WO
218

(2)

THE ANAESTHESIA VIVA

A Primary FRCA Companion

VOLUME 2

Physics, clinical measurement, safety and clinical anaesthesia

Second Edition

WITHDRAWN

D0318034

The Anaesthesia Viva

VOLUME 2
Physics, Clinical Measurement, Safety & Clinical Anaesthesia

Second Edition

Mark Blunt

John Urquhart

Colin Pinnock

With contributions from Carol Chong

WITHDRAWN

GMM

London ◆ San Francisco

\\(G\M\M\)

© 2004
Greenwich Medical Media Ltd
137 Euston Road
London
NW1 2AA

ISBN 1841101036

This Edition First Published 2003

First Edition Published 1996
Reprinted 1997, 2001, 2004 (twice).

Apart from any fair dealing for the purposes of research or private study, or criticism or review, as permitted under the UK Copyright Designs and Patents Act, 1988, this publication may not be reproduced, stored, or transmitted, in any form or by any means, without the prior permission in writing of the publishers, or in the case of reprographic reproduction only in accordance with the terms of the licences issued by the Copyright Licensing Agency in the UK, or in accordance with the terms of the licences issued by the appropriate Reproduction Rights Organization outside the UK. Enquiries concerning reproduction outside the terms stated here should be sent to the publishers at the London address printed above.

The publisher makes no representation, express or implied, with regard to the accuracy of the information contained in this book and cannot accept any legal responsibility or liability for any errors or ommissions that may be made.

The rights of Mark Blunt, John Urquhart and Colin Pinnock to be identified as authors of this work have been asserted by them in accordance with the Copyright, Designs and Patents Act 1988.

A catalogue record for this book is available from the British Library

Produced and Designed by
Saxon Graphics Limited, Derby

Printed by Cromwell Press, Trowbridge, UK

Foreword to the First Edition

1996 has seen a fundamental change in postgraduate training of anaesthetists. In place of the traditional 'apprentice system' without a clear start and finish there is now a structured course of training, under the auspices of the Royal College of Anaesthetists, consisting of two years at Senior House Officer (SHO) level and four years as a specialist registrar (SpR) with a new two part examination (Primary and Final) for the Diploma of Fellowship of the Royal College of Anaesthetists (FRCA). The new Primary examination consists of three elements, multiple choice questions (MCQs), a set of sixteen objectively structured clinical examinations (OSCEs) and two Vivas. Viva One covers physiology, pharmacology and statistics and Viva Two covers physics, clinical measurement, safety and clinical anaesthesia. The Royal College of Anaesthetists regulations allow an SHO to sit the Primary examination after twelve months of approved training, although eighteen months is recommended. Success in the Primary examination along with two satisfactory years of SHO anaesthesia training allow a trainee to apply for a ScR appointment and thus embark on a career as a specialist anaesthetist. In today's education jargon, the Primary examination is the summative assessment to complement the formative assessments carried out during the SHO years. In a sense, therefore, the Primary examination may be viewed as a screen for potential consultant anaesthetists in the future. An additional important point in the Royal College of Anaesthetists' regulations is that trainees are only allowed four attempts at each part of the FRCA. It is therefore essential that candidates for the examinations are well prepared and do not attempt the examinations until ready. How to prepare?

It is usually accepted that success in MCQs is primarily a test of core knowledge with a little technique related to understanding negative marking. Such core knowledge has to be acquired by regular reading of any of the standard large textbooks of anaesthesia, attendance at lectures and courses and perusal of the relevant specialist journals. Experience of the OSCEs from its introduction into the Part Three of the old FRCA indicated that clinical experience and practice in mock OSCEs were needed for success in this section of the examination. This leaves the Vivas. Clearly core knowledge is also needed for this type of examination as well as practice with mock events. However these may not be sufficient. The vivas consist of 'structured questions'. This means that all candidates at a particular viva session, in the interests of fairness and to avoid examiner bias, are asked the same questions. In addition, questions are reused, if they prove to be discriminating, at subsequent examinations. Inevitably a 'structured answer' begins to emerge for the successful questions. One might think that remembering questions might help subsequent examinees! However there is a large bank of questions and in addition many studies have shown that the way a candidate answers a viva question in front of the examiners is just as important as the actual knowledge. Nevertheless the concept of a structured way of considering viva questions is important. How is this to be done?

Mark Blunt and John Urquhart have brought together the disparate information needed to address the topics of Viva Two of the Primary FRCA. This book is not intended to be absolutely all encompassing – indeed such a work would probably be incomprehensible. It does however, lay out the topics in a logical order, and indicate the structures required for a candidate to answer the questions correctly. To be successful at a viva one needs to appear confident, but not *too* confident, listen carefully to the questions, speak up (the ambient noise level at viva sessions is often high and the examiners may have difficulty in hearing your answer), answer only what is asked and structure your answer in a logical order and be well prepared. The latter point is the most important, particularly in the light of the limited number of attempts now allowed at the FRCA. For the trainee, as part of your preparation for the Primary FRCA, this book and its companion volume (Urquhart JC and Blunt MC *The Anaesthesia Viva: Volume 1*) will give you the necessary starting position for the knowledge required to pass the examination.

Those of us engaged in busy consultant clinical practice or inhabiting the mythical 'ivory towers', for whom examinations are but a distant memory, might be forgiven for thinking a book such as this has little relevance to our day to day activities. However, regardless of where we practice there is always the potential embarrassment of the question we cannot answer. Indeed it is often the simplest ones which are most difficult. Study of this book will help to avoid such events and may well improve our clinical practice to the potential benefit of our patients.

Leo Strunin
BOC Professor of Anaesthesia
Director Anaesthetics Unit
Saint Bartholomew's and
The Royal London School of Medicine and Dentistry
Queen Mary's and West Field College
University of London

Preface to the Second Editions of The Anaesthesia Viva Volumes 1 and 2

It was a genuine pleasure to be invited to edit the text produced by Blunt and Urquhart from 1996. The two *viva* books have justly become popular with candidates and teachers alike due to their helpful and succinct style.

The primary examination has changed and evolved over the last few years and thus an opportunity to re-work the text appeared.

I have therefore removed question matter that no longer appears in the examination and incorporated new material from the original authors. A substantial amount of my own new material has been added and I have edited every question to maximise its suitability for revision.

There are appendices of quick reference material in each subject area which I hope will prove useful to candidates who like to have reading matter to hand in those irksome minutes before entering the *viva* hall.

I am grateful to my three co-editors of *Fundamentals of Anaesthesia*, Ted Lin, Tim Smith and Robert Jones for permission to use diagrams and annotations from that book.

In summary, I believe that these two *viva* companions will build on the success of the first editions and prove helpful to the hard working candidates.

Colin Pinnock
Alexandra Hospital, Redditch
January 2003

CONTENTS

PHYSICS, CLINICAL MEASUREMENT AND SAFETY

QUESTIONS ON PHYSICS

1. WHAT ARE THE PHYSICAL PRINCIPLES OF A 'ROTAMETER'?

> ⊃ A 'rotameter' is a variable-orifice flowmeter that allows a continuous indication of gas flow.

Within the rotameter a bobbin is supported by the gas flow within the conical glass tube. As the flow increases the bobbin rises so there is more space around the bobbin. Thus the bobbin is suspended with a variable orifice around it, and the size of the orifice therefore depends on the gas flow. The pressure drop across the bobbin is constant and equal to the weight (mass × gravity) of the bobbin divided by the cross sectional area of its base. The area of the ring around the bobbin increases as the bobbin rises, so as the flow increases the pressure drop across the bobbin remains constant.

The flow around the bobbin is a mixture of laminar and turbulent flow, due to the complex shape of the orifice. At low flows the area of the orifice is small, and it behaves like a thin tube, with the flow being more laminar, whereas higher up the area is larger relative to the length of the bobbin, and it behaves more like a short constriction in a tube, so the flow is more turbulent. Each rotameter is calibrated for the specific gas that it will measure.

In order for the rotameter to be accurate it must be vertical to prevent the bobbin touching the sides of the tube and sticking. The bobbin has fins cut into its upper surface to make it spin, and so reduce the risk of sticking due to build up of static or dirt. There is also a conductive strip or coating on the inside of the tube to reduce the build-up of electrostatic charges.

Thus, in principle, the rotameter is best described as a 'variable orifice – constant pressure drop' device.

2. WHAT IS NATURAL (RESONANT) FREQUENCY AND MECHANICAL DAMPING?

> ⊃ Damping is the tendency of a system to resist the oscillations caused by a sudden change.

Mechanical damping (as opposed to electrical damping) is mainly seen in clinical practice in direct intravascular pressure measurements. The system used consists of a column of liquid (normally dextrose, though in the case of pulmonary artery wedge pressure reading this is a column of blood then a column of dextrose), connected to a transducer. This allows changes in pressure to be detected by movement of the column of fluid that acts as a piston on the transducer that then records the movement either using a displacement or strain gauge. The resulting signal is amplified and displayed as a waveform and a digital readout.

If a sudden stepwise fall in pressure is applied to this system (e.g. after flushing the cannula) it acts in much the same way as a weight suspended on a spring and there is a tendency for oscillations to continue in the system. These oscillations occur at a consistent frequency known as the 'resonant frequency' or the 'undamped natural frequency'. Damping is a measure of the ability of the system to suppress these oscillations. In an underdamped system the oscillations continue for a long time. In an overdamped system changes occur slowly but with no overshoot. A system is said to be critically damped (D = 1.0) when there is a rapid fall in the pressure but overshoot is just avoided.

If a waveform is applied at constant amplitude but gradually increasing frequency, then as the frequency approaches the natural frequency, the amplitude recorded is increased. Then, as the frequency increases beyond the natural frequency, the recorded amplitude falls to zero. The natural frequency therefore adds inaccuracy to the system and attempts are made to increase the natural frequency until it is higher than the operating frequency of the system. In the case of a direct arterial monitor, this is about 20 Hz. It is very difficult to keep the natural frequency from imposing on the recorded frequencies in practice, as this requires short, stiff-walled, wide catheters with no connections and no air bubbles. It is therefore important to keep the distortion to a minimum and this is the function of the damping incorporated in the system.

If the system is overdamped, then it is slow to respond to changes, although overshoot will be avoided. Slow response is not desirable in a clinical system as the waveform generated is flattened and has falsely low systolic and falsely high diastolic pressures (*note though that the mean is correct*). If the system is underdamped, then there is overshoot and falsely high systolic and low diastolic pressures (due to the artefactual increase in the amplitude of the high frequency part of the curve). In fact, critical damping is normally too much for clinical applications and a better result is found when D = 0.64 (known as optimum damping).

Overdamping is frequently seen in clinical systems due to the elasticity of the walls of the tubing, the presence of air bubbles in the system or clots within the cannula, and these should be avoided.

---

3. WHAT IS A VENTURI?

> ⊃ A Venturi is a colloquial expression for a device that uses the Venturi principle, which is an application of the Bernoulli effect.

The Venturi principle states that a fluid will be entrained by the drop in pressure which results from the fluid (normally a gas) passing through a constriction, i.e. the Bernoulli effect. This is seen in nebulisers, oxygen masks, and in suction equipment remote from the central pipeline supply.

High air flow oxygen enrichment devices (HAFOE): These are a common application of the Venturi principle. (The Hudson and MC type masks are variable-performance devices, and therefore not the same as the HAFOE type). The design of the masks permit the delivery of predictable oxygen fractions according to the fresh gas flow delivered, due to the Venturi principle; in other words, the oxygen flow is entraining a known ratio of room air.

It is possible to establish the O_2 flow rate and the entrained air flow ratio for a device with the following equations:

$$100\ a \times 21\ b = 30 \times \text{required FIO}_2$$

$$a + b = 30$$

Where a = oxygen flow rate, b = entrained air flow rate, and the patient's peak inspiratory flow rate does not exceed 30 l/min.

Most HAFOE systems observe a convention of colour coding for oxygen delivery. For example:

COLOUR	DELIVERED O_2%	FRESH GAS FLOW (L/MIN)
Blue	24%	2
White	28%	4
Orange	31%	6
Yellow	35%	8
Red	40%	10
Green	60%	15

Giovanni Venturi was an Italian physicist who died in 1822.

----

4. WHAT IS THE BERNOULLI EFFECT?

> ⊃ The Bernoulli effect describes the way that fluid passes faster through a constriction, gaining kinetic energy, but losing potential energy and so reducing pressure. In this way, the total energy is preserved in accordance with Newtonian Law. If the Bernoulli effect is used to entrain a second fluid, this is known as the Venturi principle.

This is not the same as, but is frequently confused with, the Coanda effect. The Coanda effect is that a substance flowing in a tube is attracted to the walls of the tube, which is the physical principle underlying the design of some mechanical ventilators.

Daniel Bernoulli was a Swiss mathematician who died in 1782.

5. WHAT IS THE COANDA EFFECT?

When there is a constriction in a tube, there is a fall in the pressure of the fluid flowing through it. This is the basis of a venturi, but when the stream then flows along a solid surface (e.g. the wall of a wide tube), entrainment cannot occur against the wall, so the pressure at this point remains low and the flow tends to stick to the wall. If there are two outlets, the fluid does not evenly divide, but tends to flow down one limb or the other – the so-called 'Coanda effect'. This may explain some of the misdistribution of gases in the alveoli for example, or instances of myocardial ischaemia when there appear to be patent coronary arteries. The Coanda effect can be used to allow the control of the flow of gas down one of two tubes, by using a small volume switching flow. Once the flow is established down one of the tubes, the switching flow can be stopped and flow will continue down the appropriate tube. This is the basis of fluid logic, and can be used in ventilators to reduce the number of valves and moving parts.

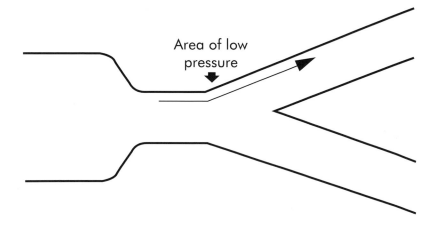

Area of low
pressure

6. DEFINE THE FOLLOWING TERMS

⊃ **Critical temperature**

⊃ **Vapour and gas**

⊃ **Critical pressure**

⊃ **Critical flow**

Critical temperature is defined as the temperature above which a substance cannot be liquefied by pressure alone.

A vapour is the term for a substance in the gaseous phase at or below its critical temperature. A gas applies to a substance that is above its critical temperature.

Critical pressure is the pressure required to liquefy a substance at its critical temperature.

Critical flow is the flow when the Reynold's number is 2000 and so the flow of the fluid is liable to change from laminar to turbulent.

Reynold's number $= \dfrac{\nu \rho d}{\eta}$

Where: ν = linear velocity of the fluid

ρ = density

d = diameter of the tube

η = viscosity

7. IN WHAT WAY DOES THE OUTPUT FROM AN 'IDEAL' VAPORISER CHANGE AT HIGH ALTITUDE AND WHY?

⊃ In general, vaporisers are designed to work by fully saturating a specific proportion of the gas flowing along the back bar.

Therefore, their output may be regarded as consisting of two separate volumes of gas; the first that has passed through the vaporiser chamber and contains anaesthetic vapour ideally at its saturated vapour pressure (SVP) and the second consisting of the gas that contains no anaesthetic vapour that has by-passed the vaporising chamber.

As the SVP of the vapour is unchanged at altitude, the partial pressure of anaesthetic agent that comes out of the vaporising chamber will be unchanged. However, the concentration of gas that leaves the chamber will be dependent on the ratio of that pressure to the total pressure (i.e. SVP : P_{atm}). As the splitting ratio will be the same (it is this that the dial on the vaporiser changes), the concentration in the gas leaving the vaporiser will be changed inversely to the change in P_{atm}.

So, if:

P_{sea} = atmospheric pressure at sea level

P_{alt} = atmospheric pressure at altitude

C = concentration at sea level

C' = concentration at altitude

$$C' = C \times \frac{P_{sea}}{P_{alt}}$$

Therefore, as the altitude increases and the barometric pressure falls, the concentration from the vaporiser rises.

BUT the effect of the vapour does not depend on the concentration but on the partial pressure of the vapour. This has not changed, so the effect of using a vaporiser that is calibrated at sea level at the setting that one would normally use is the same. In fact, in a normal vaporiser, there are slight differences because the gas entering the vaporiser has a lower density, so the resistance from the high-resistance pathway through the vaporising chamber is slightly less. The vapour pressure in the chamber will therefore tend to approach SVP more fully and so the partial pressure of vapour will be higher.

The above description applies to current plenum vaporiser types (e.g. TEC series). Direct injection vaporisers, such as those used for Desflurane, are designed around different physical principles.

___

8. WHAT IS THE DIFFERENCE BETWEEN ABSOLUTE AND GAUGE PRESSURE?

⊃ **Consider two tubes of mercury.**

Absolute pressure is most easily visualised as the height of a column of fluid that the pressure will support (though it should be noted that pressure is now strictly defined in terms of force per unit area). Absolute pressure is measured with respect to zero pressure (a vacuum). On the other hand, gauge pressure is the pressure above or below atmospheric pressure. The two pressures may be visualised thus:

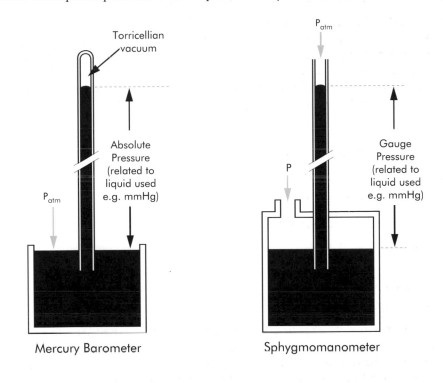

Mercury Barometer   Sphygmomanometer

9. WHAT WOULD HAPPEN TO THE MENISCUS OF A MERCURY MANOMETER IF A FEW DROPS OF ISOFLURANE WERE INTRODUCED INTO THE VACUUM ABOVE IT?

⊃ **This is a complicated sounding question that merely tests the understanding of some very simple physical principles – pressure and saturated vapour pressure.**

Atmospheric pressure (at sea level and room temperature) will support a column of mercury 760 mm high in a liquid manometer. If a small amount of any liquid is introduced into the vacuum above there will be a pressure exerted on the top of the mercury column that is equal to the saturated vapour pressure of that vapour at room temperature. Thus the meniscus will fall so that the height of the column is equal to:

Height $= P_{atm} - SVP_{liquid}$

Thus, in this instance:

Height $=$ 760 mm – 250 mm

$=$ 510 mm

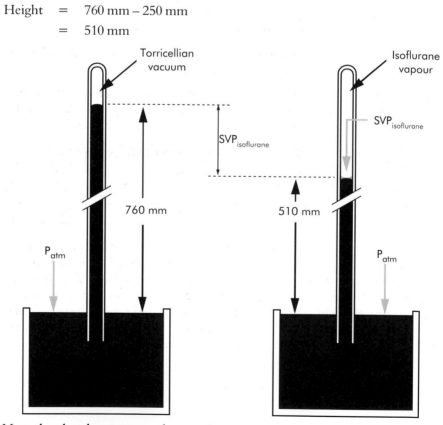

Note also that the answer to the question:

"What is present in the Torricellian vacuum?" is: Mercury vapour at SVP_{Hg}

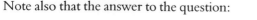

10. WHAT IS 'FILLING RATIO' AND WHY SHOULD IT BE LESS THAN 1.0?

> ⊃ A cylinder containing only gas can be easily filled to a set point by measuring the pressure in the cylinder. However, one containing liquid needs another method to assess adequacy of filling and avoid overfilling.

Because a cylinder of nitrous oxide contains liquid and vapour with a pressure equal to the SVP of nitrous oxide at the ambient temperature, it is impossible to tell the amount of N_2O within the cylinder. This is in contrast to oxygen, which remains as a compressed gas. In the latter case, the amount of O_2 within the cylinder is equal to the absolute pressure of the cylinder contents in atmospheres × the volume of the cylinder. In order to measure the contents of a N_2O cylinder it is necessary to weigh the cylinder and subtract the mass of the empty cylinder. To equate this to a guide of the size of the cylinder and thus give an 'average density' of the contents, this is divided by the mass of water the cylinder would hold:

$$\text{Filling Ratio} = \frac{\text{Mass of nitrous oxide in the cylinder}}{\text{Mass of water that the cylinder would hold}}$$

In our temperate climate, the maximum permissible filling ratio is 0.75 though here, as in tropical regions, the most commonly used value is 0.67.

Considering the pressure within a cylinder at various temperatures at the normal filling ratio of 0.67 and comparing it with the pressure at a ratio of 0.77, where the cylinder at 20°C is almost totally full of liquid, the following can be seen:

FILLING RATIO	PRESSURE AT VARIOUS TEMPERATURES (BAR)		
	20°C	40°C	60°C
0.67	51	90	160
0.77	51	125	190

Thus, the pressure at 40°C (above the critical temperature and hence with the cylinder containing only gas) has risen to 90 bar for the normal filling but is already approaching the pressure within an oxygen cylinder for the 'overfilled' cylinder. This is a temperature that is rare in the UK but is common in the tropics. However, at 60°C the pressure of the normal cylinder has risen to 160 bar (approximately the same as a 'full' oxygen cylinder at the same temperature), but the 'overfilled' cylinder is at 190 bar and rapidly approaching the testing pressure of the cylinder, above which it may explode.

---

11. HOW DOES A PRESSURE REGULATOR WORK?

> ⊃ **A diagram is invaluable in answering this question.**

The high pressure inside gas cylinders is reduced by a pressure regulator before connection to equipment such as an anaesthetic machine. An example of a single stage regulator which might be used to reduce oxygen cylinder pressure from 13 700 kPa to 420 kPa is shown below. Cylinder pressure (P) is reduced to the supply pressure (p) as oxygen passes through the small inlet valve (area = a) into the control chamber. The pressure in the control chamber (p) is controlled by a compression spring acting on a diaphragm (area = A) which is coupled mechanically to the inlet valve. The supply pressure is thus controlled by the force (F) in the spring. This can be expressed by the following equation;

$$F = \text{Force acting on conical valve} + \text{Force acting on diaphragm}$$

$$= Pa + pA$$

If it is assumed that the force in the spring remains constant (i.e. the range of movement in the spring is small compared to its total length), then any change in the supply or cylinder pressures will cause a compensating change as the diaphragm moves and varies the effective area of the inlet valve. In the above equation, if F is constant, a decrease in pA (drop in supply pressure due to increased demand) causes an increase in Pa (increased flow from cylinder). Alternatively, if Pa decreases (due to cylinder pressure falling as it empties), pA will increase (due to increased flow from cylinder).

Thus, the pressure regulator not only reduces the cylinder pressure to a suitable supply pressure but, also compensates for changes in demand or cylinder pressure. The sensitivity of this control depends on the ratio of the area diaphragm to the area of the valve, (which is usually 200: 1).

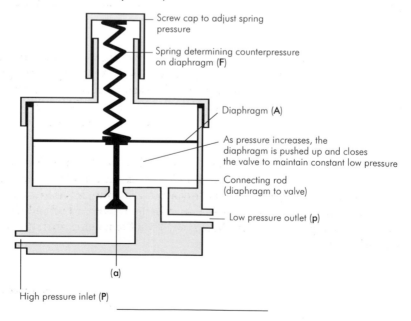

Screw cap to adjust spring pressure

Spring determining counterpressure on diaphragm (**F**)

Diaphragm (**A**)

As pressure increases, the diaphragm is pushed up and closes the valve to maintain constant low pressure

Connecting rod (diaphragm to valve)

Low pressure outlet (**p**)

(**a**)

High pressure inlet (**P**)

12. WHAT HAPPENS TO THE PRESSURE WITHIN A NITROUS OXIDE CYLINDER AS IT IS DISCHARGED?

> ⊃ At room temperature, nitrous oxide is below its critical temperature, and so the nitrous oxide cylinder contains both liquid and vapour under pressure. The pressure within the cylinder is therefore the saturated vapour pressure of N_2O at room temperature.

The pressure is initially 52 bar, and the cylinder will contain vapour at its SVP whilst there is still some liquid remaining within it, with liquid vaporising to maintain the pressure as vapour is released from the cylinder. Once the amount of N_2O within the cylinder has fallen to such an extent that all the liquid has vaporised, the pressure within the cylinder falls as the vapour is released. Therefore, it may be assumed that the pressure within the cylinder will fall thus:

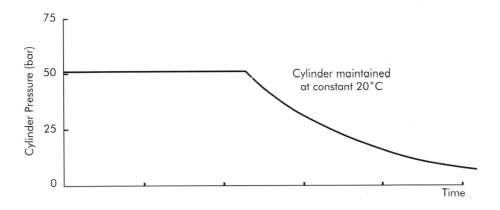

In fact, this is not the case in practice because as the liquid vaporises it requires energy to overcome the latent heat of vaporisation, and this energy is supplied by heat from the N_2O itself, the cylinder and the surrounding air. Therefore, the temperature of the liquid N_2O falls. This is why the outside of the cylinder is seen to condense water vapour and even to be covered with frost when the cylinder is in use.

The pressure within the cylinder remains at the SVP of N_2O. This falls with falling temperature, so the pressure within the cylinder falls as the cylinder is continuously discharged. In fact, if a 900 l cylinder is discharged at 8 l/min, it is impossible to see when the liquid is exhausted. However, if the cylinder is switched off and allowed to return to room temperature whilst there is still liquid remaining, then the pressure will return to 52 bar.

continued overleaf

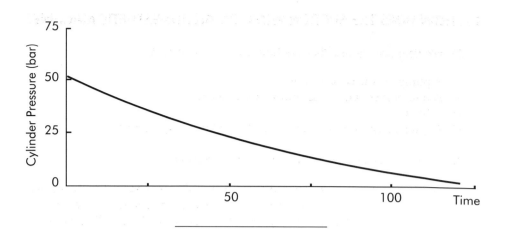

13. WHAT IS MEANT BY BOILING? WHAT IS LATENT HEAT OF VAPORISATION?

> ⊃ These two topics are often asked together as linked concepts.

Boiling is the process whereby a substance is converted from its liquid to its vapour phase. What happens is that bubbles of vapour form and then escape from the surface of the liquid. Obviously, the pressure within the bubble is opposed by the tension at the surface, which tends to stop the bubble escaping from the liquid. If the vapour pressure is equal to or greater than the pressure on the surface (i.e. the saturated vapour pressure is equal to or greater than the external pressure, commonly the atmospheric pressure) then the bubble is likely to escape and boiling occurs. The temperature at which the SVP equals the ambient pressure is the temperature at which boiling occurs (by convention the 'boiling point' is the temperature at which SVP equals 1 atmosphere – 760 mmHg).

Latent heat of vaporisation is the energy required to fuel this process and convert a unit mass of liquid from the liquid phase to the vapour phase, at a constant temperature and at a specified pressure. At lower pressures (and therefore lower temperatures) the latent heat of vaporisation is larger.

14. HOW DOES THE SUCTION WORK ON AN ANAESTHETIC MACHINE?

⊃ Medical devices usually have four central components:

- A pump or source of vacuum
- A reservoir containing an anti-foaming agent
- A filter
- A gauge, reading anticlockwise, with a yellow background

⊃ Suction may be delivered by one of three methods:

- Mechanical means – foot pump or hand-held device, both of which operate on a piston principle; these are used in field locations and for resuscitation.
- Venturi, employing a gas supply (usually oxygen) – this is usually used at locations where there is no central vacuum system, such as operating theatres in hospitals with no pipeline gases. Gases are supplied from cylinders and suction is therefore driven by these gases. This is an expensive way of providing suction, as it consumes 20 l/min from the gas supply.
- Central vacuum supply, which is the commonest system in theatre and the one you should be able to describe.

The source of suction is a pump (usually two) located centrally, which eliminates filtered gas to the atmosphere. This must be capable of sustaining a vacuum of not less than 400 mmHg below atmospheric pressure. There is a reservoir, which is protected by bacterial filters. The pipelines emerge from the wall alongside piped gas supplies at a Schrader valve, which is colour-coded yellow (in the UK) as is the pipeline within the theatre. The standard for anaesthetic purposes is that it should take no more than 10 seconds to generate -500 mmHg, with a displacement capacity of 25 l/min. The tubing needs to have low resistance and low compliance.

Use a diagram to illustrate these points:

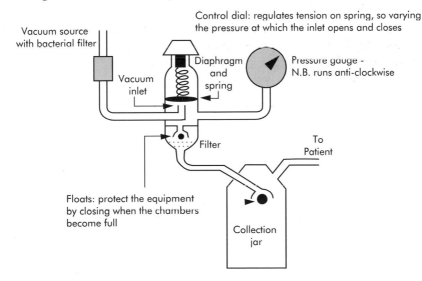

15

15. WHAT IS THE DIFFERENCE BETWEEN DIFFERENT TYPES OF DIATHERMY?

⊃ Diathermy is the passage of an electrical current through tissue, generating heat, in order to either coagulate blood vessels or cut through tissue, or both.

⊃ The key expression when discussing diathermy is *current density*. With unipolar diathermy, when the current passes through the diathermy plate on the patient, there is a wide area exposed to the current and the heating effect is minimal. At the forceps, however, the area exposed to the current and through which that current passes is very small, and the current density is therefore high; the heat generated is therefore considerable.

The current is of high frequency, 500 KHz – 1.5 MHz (Mains supply is 50 Hz).

Cutting diathermy – This uses current in an alternating sine-wave pattern.

Coagulation diathermy – This uses current in a pulsed, sine wave pattern.

Unipolar diathermy – The forceps represent one electrode, the plate on the patient the other.

Bipolar diathermy – Current passes between the two blades of a forceps; no plate is required. This form is safer in the presence of a pacemaker. However, only 40 Watts of energy can be delivered using bipolar diathermy, as opposed to 150 – 400 Watts with unipolar diathermy.

---

16. WHAT PROBLEMS MAY OCCUR FROM THE USE OF DIATHERMY?

⊃ **Injuries arising from the misuse of diathermy represent an ongoing source of litigation.**

The problems may be listed as follows:

Burns

■ Incorrect siting of the plate when using unipolar diathermy, with arcing and skin burns because of increased current density.

■ Ignition of skin preparation spirit – some types burn with an invisible flame.

■ Inadvertent activation of diathermy while forceps is in contact with tissue remote from the operative site. This is why the forceps are kept in an insulated holder and a buzzer sounded to indicate operation of the diathermy.

■ Activation of the diathermy in contact with a metal object, which in turn is in contact with the patient and remote from the operative site.

Earthing

In certain machines, the plate will be earthed. If this is the case, and it is not properly applied, or if the connections to it are faulty, then current may go to earth by other routes. These include the ECG machine via the electrodes and metal drip poles. Because current density at these sites is high, burns will result. Newer machines do not have earthed plates.

Pacemakers

Unipolar diathermy may destabilise pacemakers, especially if the current traverses the chest. Recommendations for the use of diathermy with pacemakers are summarised below.

Recommendations for the use of diathermy with pacemakers
■ Place the indifferent electrode on the same side as the operation and as far from the pacemaker unit as possible
■ Limit the use of diathermy as much as possible
■ Use the lowest current setting possible
■ Use bipolar diathermy (but power of coagulation is less)
■ Monitor patient ECG constantly
■ Keep the pacemaker programmer available, where appropriate

Monitoring

Activation of diathermy interferes with monitoring, especially with pulse oximetry and, to a lesser extent, with ECG.

17. WHAT DOES A TRANSDUCER DO?

⊃ This is a frequent question. Regrettably it is all too often answered badly – usually with a 'woolly' definition.

⊃ A transducer is quite simply a device that converts one form of energy into another, for the purposes of measurement. The second form of energy is normally electrical.

A pressure transducer measures, indirectly, the pressure in the circulation, in a breathing system, or an infusion device. It consists of a semiconductor, whose shape is deformed by the action of the pressure in proportion to the pressure applied, altering its conductivity. Arterial pressure transducers most commonly utilise a strain gauge principle where the deformation of a diaphragm with incorporated electrical resistance alters its conductivity and although circuitry is now integrated, the Wheatstone bridge calculation still applies.

18. WHAT IS A WHEATSTONE BRIDGE?

⊃ Many transducers used in medical practice depend on a physical change causing a change in their resistance. A Wheatstone bridge is a special arrangement of resistors designed to amplify this change in resistance.

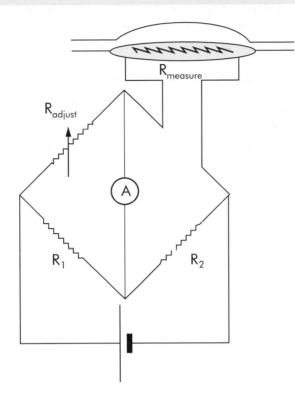

The simplest form of the Wheatstone bridge is designed so that it is balanced and there is no flow of current from one side to the other (i.e. the ammeter reads zero). This balance is achieved by adjusting the resistance in the adjustment leg to compensate for the change in the measurement leg. The resistance can then be calculated by:

$$\frac{R_{measure}}{R_{adjust}} = \frac{R_2}{R_1}$$

In practice, however, the current flow across the bridge is amplified and this is measured or displayed. Furthermore if **all** the resistances are part of the transducer (e.g. a strain gauge used to measure deflection of a diaphragm due to pressure) and these are set up so that two resistances increase whilst the other two decrease with the change in strain, the electrical signal is amplified.

19. WHAT IS A CAPACITOR? GIVE AN EXAMPLE OF ITS IMPORTANCE IN PRACTICE.

> ⊃ **A capacitor is a body that is able to hold electrical charge. It consists of two conductive plates separated by an insulator (dielectric medium). Capacitance is a measure of that ability.**

The capacitor most frequently encountered in medical practice is the defibrillator. In this device, the capacitor is placed in a switched part of the circuit so that it may be 'charged' by applying a voltage across the two plates and allowing the build up of charge. The voltage is considerably higher than mains voltage and this is achieved using a transformer. When the charging reaches a predetermined point, the voltage is switched off but the charge in the capacitor remains. When the circuit is switched to 'defibrillate' this charge is released as a pulse of current (since current is merely charge delivered per second), initially at the potential difference (i.e. voltage) that was present when the capacitor was charged. The circuit generally has an inductor to prolong the duration of the current flow. This duration is typically about 3 msec. The current flowing for that short time is in the order of 32 A, initially at about 5000 V. The energy supplied can be derived from the charge stored multiplied by the mean voltage (i.e. half the charging voltage).

You will be expected to be able to draw the circuit as shown below.

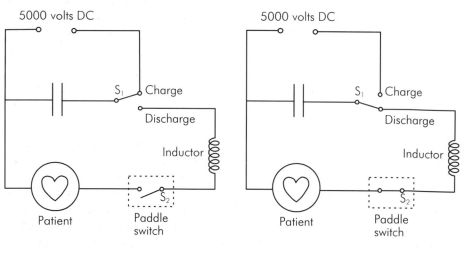

(a) Defibrillator charging

(b) Defibrillator discharging

20. WHAT IS IMPEDANCE AND WHEN IS IT OF VALUE IN MEDICAL MEASUREMENT?

> ⟳ **Impedance is a measure of the obstruction to current flow through a capacitor.**

The resistance to current flow through a capacitor is not constant. When a DC circuit is switched on, the current flowing through the capacitor rapidly falls to zero (by an exponential decline), and the potential difference (the voltage) across the capacitor rises. In an AC circuit, the current is being continually switched on and off, and the capacitor does not reach a steady state. The current flow through the capacitor follows the voltage change but is 90° out of phase.

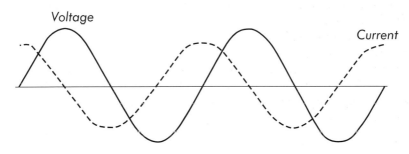

The current flow through the capacitor is proportional not to the voltage itself but to the rate of change of the voltage (dV/dt), and so is related to the frequency of the AC supply. As the current varies with frequency, it is reasonable to assume that the hindrance to the current flow will change with frequency. This is termed the 'reactance' of the capacitor and it is inversely proportional to the frequency of the supply.

The circuit will also have a resistance (constant hindrance to flow that is not frequency dependent) and the resistance and the reactance are taken together to find the opposition to flow of the capacitance circuit. This is called the impedance and is quoted at a particular frequency.

All tissues of the body can act as capacitors and have impedance. Furthermore this impedance is related to the constituents of that tissue, so if those constituents change, the impedance changes. Thus, if the tissue between two electrodes contains increased blood (due to vasodilation) then the impedance will change. Another example is that an increase in the air in the chest changes the thoracic impedance. Although the absolute value of the impedance is widely variable, the change in value is relatively linear and the voltage change across the electrodes can be calibrated (in the latter case using expired spirometry for an initial calibration). This can be used as a rapid-responding non-invasive measure of ventilation. Other uses include measurement of stroke volume in a beat-to-beat manner.

21. WHAT ARE THE PRINCIPLE COMPONENTS OF A SCAVENGING SYSTEM?

⊃ **A scavenging system is a group of components designed to transfer waste anaesthetic gases from the breathing system to a safe remote location.**

All scavenging systems consist of:

- A collecting device – a shroud around the exhaust valve, or a canopy over a recovering patient, although the latter is a rarity.
- A means of taking the gases away using tubing – scavenging connections are 30 mm diameter, to prevent inadvertent connection to the breathing system.
- A receiving system (a reservoir of some description) – a pressure relief valve is usual to prevent the possibility of barotrauma.
- An exhaust system to discharge the gases safely.

Passage of gases through the systems may be powered either by the patient's expiration (passive systems) or by active means.

Passive scavenging

This may be a simple tube leading out to atmosphere. The Cardiff Aldasorber is a canister of activated charcoal connected to the exhaust tubing, and extracts volatile anaesthetic agents but not N_2O. It weighs 1 kg when new and this allows calculation of the extent of its use and of the time at which it should be replaced.

Active scavenging

This is able to cope better with the variation in gas flow rates that are seen in normal anaesthetic practice, and normally consists of a type of fan system that produces a constant low suction pressure (sub-anaesthetic pressure). Pipeline suction is inappropriate because a low-pressure system is needed for safety reasons. The source should remove 75 l/min. Other methods of driving scavenging systems include venturi systems.

The gases are collected and then ducted to a collecting system that must contain some form of reservoir, either a reservoir bag or an open-ended vessel. If this is a closed vessel, then there should be a high-pressure valve (10 cmH$_2$O) to avoid backflow of gases if the capacity is exceeded or there is a blockage. It also needs a low-pressure valve (-0.5 cmH$_2$O) to allow air in when the expired gas flow does not meet the disposal system demands. These are unnecessary if an open vessel is used, as this effectively provides them via the opening. An air-break is often used to achieve this in modern systems. The exhaust system should then discharge the gases outside at a suitable site away from areas where personnel are working.

PASSIVE SCAVENGING

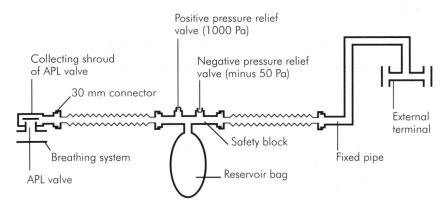

Positive pressure relief valve (1000 Pa)

Collecting shroud of APL valve

Negative pressure relief valve (minus 50 Pa)

30 mm connector

External terminal

Breathing system

Safety block

Fixed pipe

APL valve

Reservoir bag

ACTIVE SCAVENGING

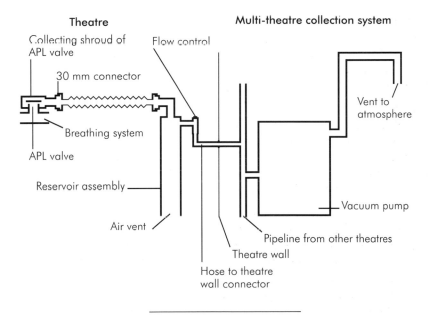

Theatre

Multi-theatre collection system

Collecting shroud of APL valve

Flow control

30 mm connector

Vent to atmosphere

Breathing system

APL valve

Reservoir assembly

Vacuum pump

Air vent

Pipeline from other theatres

Theatre wall

Hose to theatre wall connector

22. WHAT IS MICROSHOCK AND HOW IS IT PREVENTED?

> ⊃ The risk of ventricular fibrillation relates to the current density in the heart so a very small voltage within the heart can be just as lethal as a much larger one applied to the skin of a hand.

It is well known that the passage of an electrical current through the heart may lead to ventricular fibrillation. If the electrical current comes from touching a live wire with a hand and the current passes to earth via the feet, most of that current passes through the non-cardiac tissues of the trunk, with only a small proportion passing through the heart. Thus, a relatively large current is required to cause ventricular fibrillation. However, if the current comes from an intracardiac catheter, then almost all of the current will pass through the heart. In this case only a very small current is required to cause ventricular fibrillation (in the order of 150 μA). It should also be noted that as the current density is increased, the voltage similarly can be reduced, so it is possible to get microshock with battery voltages (12 V) or less.

Some potential sources of microshock are:
- Central venous catheter
- Pulmonary artery catheter
- Temporary external pacemaker
- Oesophageal temperature probe in lower third of oesophagus
- Statically-charged staff touching any of the above

Prevention of microshock:
- Use appropriate equipment in good order. Equipment specifications may refer to leakage current generation and the risk of microshock. For example:
  CF (Cardiac, floating) – leakage <50 μA through cardiac connection.
  BF (Non cardiac, floating) – leakage <500 μA through patient connection with single fault
- Choose suitable footwear to optimise impedance
- Use antistatic flooring
- Use an isolated patient circuit – with no earth connection to patient
- Ensure optimum design of earthing circuits for equipment
- Ensure correct humidity in theatre

23. WHICH CAN PRODUCE A HIGHER PRESSURE ON INJECTION – A 2 ml OR 20 ml SYRINGE?

> ⊃ The pressure of the injecting liquid is dependent on the force exerted on the syringe and the area over which that force acts.

Assuming the same force is applied, this question asks for knowledge of a fundamental principle.

$$P = \frac{f}{a}$$

P = pressure developed

f = force of injection

a = cross-sectional area

The smaller the cross-sectional area, the higher the pressure developed, and the answer to the question is that the 2 ml syringe allows the higher pressure to be developed.

———————————

24. WHAT ARE THE BASIC SI UNITS?

⊃ The Système Internationale units were introduced by the General Conference on Weights and Measures in 1960 and are based on the Metric system. There are base units and derived units.

Base units:

UNIT	UNIT OF:	DEFINITION
Metre	Length	The distance occupied by 1,650,763.73 wavelengths of light from gaseous krypton. The original bar of platinum–iridium against which the metre was calibrated ceased to be used after concerns about its consistent length over time
Second	Time	The definition relates to the frequency of radiation emitted by ^{133}Caesium It is also roughly $1 \div 24 \times 60 \times 60$ of the time taken for earth to complete one revolution.
Kilogram	Mass	There is a standard cylinder of platinum–iridium against which the kilogram is calibrated. It is about 37 mm in each dimension and is kept near Paris.
Ampere	Electric current	The current in two straight parallel wires 1 metre apart in a vacuum which will produce a force of 2×10^7 Newtons/metre on each of the wires.
Kelvin	Temperature	0°K is −273.16°C. The exact definition is: $1K = 1/273.16$ of the thermodynamic scale temperature of the triple point of water, where water in sold, liquid and gaseous state are in equilibrium
Candela	Luminous intensity	Involves the intensity of a body at the freezing point of platinum
Mole	Substance	The quantity of a substance containing Avogadro's number of particles (6.022×10^{23}), the number of particles as atoms in 12 grams of ^{12}Carbon.

Derived units:

UNIT	UNIT OF:	DEFINITION
Newton	Force	Force = mass × acceleration. 1 Newton = the force required to accelerate a mass of 1 kg by 1 m/s^2
Pascal	Pressure	Pressure = force / area 1 Pascal = 1 N/m^2
Joule	Energy, work	Potential energy is the energy possessed by a body because of its position; kinetic energy is the energy of a body due to its motion. 1 Joule is the work done (energy used) when a force of 1 N moves 1 metre
Watt	Power	Power is the rate of doing work, = work/time. 1 Watt = 1 joule/second
Hertz	Frequency	1 Hertz = 1 cycle/second

Newton's 3 Laws of Motion:

- A body continues in its state of rest or in its uniform motion in a straight line unless acted upon by an external force.
- When a force acts on a body, the rate of change of momentum in the body is proportional to the force and is in the same direction as that in which the force acts.
- For every action there is an equal and opposite reaction.

The law of conservation of energy is that energy can be neither created nor destroyed, but only transformed from one state to another.

---

25. HOW DOES A LASER WORK?

⊃ **LASER is an acronym of L̲ight A̲mplification by S̲imulated E̲mission of R̲adiation.**

Lasers produce an intense beam of light that is monochromatic (of one wavelength). The beam is emitted as a parallel stream of photons with little or no divergence so it can be used to deliver a large amount of energy accurately to small areas of tissue.

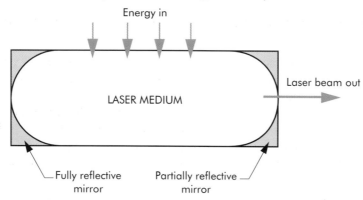

The laser works by absorbing energy from an external source (e.g. a flashlight or high-voltage discharge). This energy may then be released as a photon of a specific wavelength. If this is then reflected back into the laser medium and meets another excited atom, that atom releases its energy in the form of another photon that is parallel and in phase with the other photon. These may then cause a further similar reaction, and the resulting chain reaction leads to release of an intense form of light in phase and parallel. This is emitted from the lasing chamber and in most medical cases is directed onto the target tissue by a fibre-optic wand.

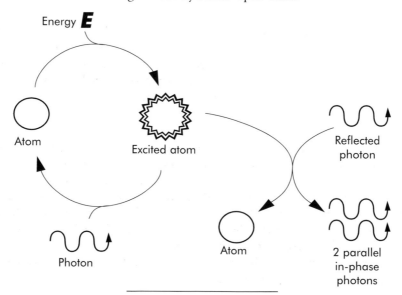

26. WHY ARE DIFFERENT LASERS USED THERAPEUTICALLY AND WHAT ARE THE GENERAL AND SPECIFIC RISKS THAT RELATE TO THE ANAESTHETIST?

⊃ **The most common lasers in therapeutic use are carbon dioxide, argon and Nd: YAG (neodymium : yttrium–aluminium garnet). A full list of applied types is given later.**

The differing media are used in order to vary the depth of penetration, the wavelength of the light and the power of the beam.

- **Carbon dioxide** light is infrared and is absorbed by water that is vaporised, destroying the tissue contents. Thus, these lasers are used as 'scalpels' to cut into tissues with haemostasis.
- **Argon** lasers produce light in the blue-green area of the visible spectrum and so are maximally absorbed by red tissues. Thus, they tend to be directed at the small vessels within the transparent tissue of the eye.
- **The Nd: YAG** laser is a near infra-red laser that is used for penetrating deeply into tissues.

The **general dangers** of laser usage are due to the non-divergent beam that therefore has almost no loss of power as the distance from the source is increased. The greatest danger is of light entering the eye where it will tend to burn the retina as well as damaging the aqueous and vitreous humours, cornea and lens. Indeed, the major danger is of light landing on the 'blind spot' and damaging the optic nerve as this can cause irreversible total blindness. Surfaces around the target tissue should be non-reflective as the dangers are compounded by reflection in glossy surfaces. The lesser danger is of damage to skin or tissues distant to the target tissue.

The **specific dangers** for anaesthetists relate to the risk of fire in the oxygen-enriched atmosphere in and around the airway. This is most commonly encountered in ENT procedures, but it should be remembered that surgical drapes could hold a high concentration of oxygen or combustion-supporting nitrous oxide that can be ignited if the laser is accidentally directed below them.

The following measures should be taken to reduce the risks:

- Flammable anaesthetic agents should not be used (including nitrous oxide).
- Laser-resistant endotracheal tubes should be used. A standard tube is highly flammable in the airway environment and will ignite if the laser beam is directed at it, and the technique of covering this with silver-foil may cause damage to the larynx or the vocal cords and may not shield the tube fully. It should however be noted that even laser-resistant disposable tubes will not withstand direct laser light for any length of time.
- Inspired oxygen should be diluted with air, ideally to an F_IO_2 of 0.25 or less, if the patient can cope with this.

■ Black-coloured instruments reduce the risk of reflections.
■ Damage to nearby tissues should be avoided by covering them with wet swabs.

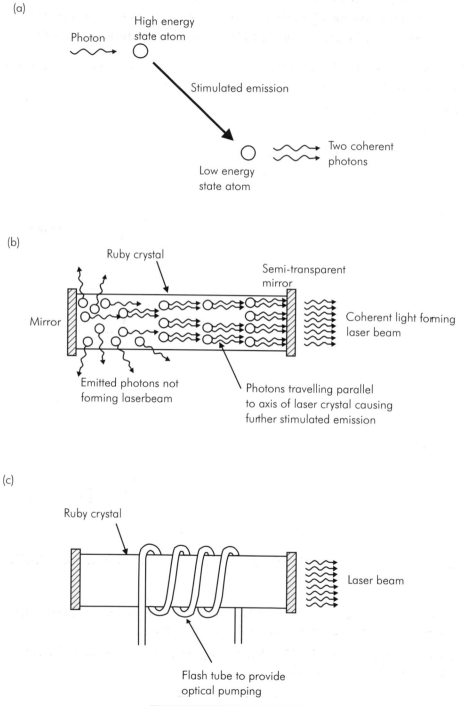

(a)

Photon

High energy state atom

Stimulated emission

Two coherent photons

Low energy state atom

(b)

Ruby crystal

Semi-transparent mirror

Mirror

Coherent light forming laser beam

Emitted photons not forming laserbeam

Photons travelling parallel to axis of laser crystal causing further stimulated emission

(c)

Ruby crystal

Laser beam

Flash tube to provide optical pumping

27. WHAT IS OHM'S LAW?

> ⊃ **This question is often followed by the application of Ohm's law in circuits and the addition of resistances and capacitances (in series and parallel) as a related topic. You may also be shown circuit symbols to identify.**

Ohm's law states that the current passing through a conductor is proportional to the potential difference across it (at a constant temperature).

This is usually expressed as:

$V = I\,R$

Ohm was a German physicist from the 1800's.

Circuit symbols to learn are shown below.

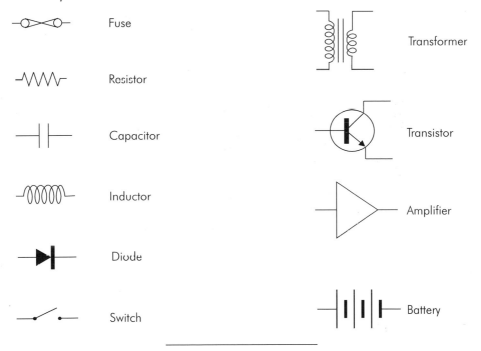

Fuse		Transformer
Resistor		
Capacitor		Transistor
Inductor		
Diode		Amplifier
Switch		Battery

28. WHAT IS MEANT BY TRIPLE POINT? WHAT IS THE TRIPLE POINT OF WATER?

The triple point of a substance is the temperature (at a certain pressure) at which the solid, liquid and vapour forms of the substance co-exist.

For water, the triple point is 273.16 Kelvin at a pressure of 611.2 Pascals. Note particularly that this defines the Kelvin.

29. DEFINE THE FOLLOWING PREFIXES TO THE POWER OF TEN.

⊃ You will most often find this question linked to the definition of SI units. A bad answer will not necessarily gain a 1 mark but it will make a bad start to the viva. A little revision time will therefore be well spent.
A frequent associated topic is the quantification of atmospheric pressure in various units (kPa, mmHg, Atm, PSI, cmH_2O etc) – be warned!

The more common prefixes that you should know are:

PREFIX	LETTER	MULTIPLYING FACTOR
Exa	E	10^{18}
Peta	P	10^{15}
tera	T	10^{12}
giga	G	10^{9}
mega	M	10^{6}
kilo	k	10^{3}
hecto	h	10^{2}
deca	da	10
deci	d	10^{-1}
centi	c	10^{-2}
milli	m	10^{-3}
micro	μ	10^{-6}
nano	n	10^{-9}
pico	p	10^{-12}
femto	f	10^{-15}
atto	a	10^{-18}

30. WHAT ARE THE DIFFERNCES BETWEEN SCALAR AND VECTOR QUANTITIES? GIVE EXAMPLES OF EACH.

⊃ A scalar quantity is defined solely by its magnitude.

Scalars include quantities such as **temperature** and **mass**.

⊃ A vector quantity requires both magnitude and direction to be defined.

Vectors include quantities such as **force**, **velocity** and **displacement** (change in position). Simple addition or subtraction of vector quantities cannot be performed without reference to their direction. Vector quantities may be added using simple geometrical rules, to give a resultant vector. So, consider the sum of a force of 1 Newton added to another force of 1 Newton. If the forces are in opposite directions the result is zero, if they act in the same direction the result is a force of 2 Newtons.

2

QUESTIONS ON CLINICAL MEASUREMENT

1. HOW DOES A pH ELECTRODE WORK?

> ⊃ The pH electrode is an ion-selective electrode that relies on the electric
> potential generated by the movement of H^+ ions between the sample
> liquid and a reference buffer at known $[H^+]$.

The sample and the buffer are separated by hydrogen-ion sensitive glass so the development of current depends on the movement of hydrogen ions alone. The buffer is in contact with a Ag/AgCl electrode and there also needs to be a reference electrode in contact with the blood. This electrode is separated from the blood by a semi-permeable membrane to avoid protein contamination and the electrode is kept in contact with the blood by a saturated potassium chloride solution.

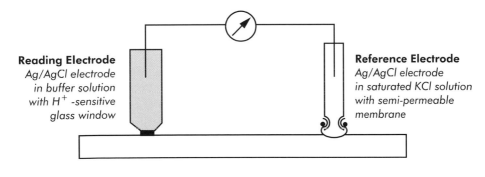

Reading Electrode
Ag/AgCl electrode
in buffer solution
with H^+-sensitive
glass window

Reference Electrode
Ag/AgCl electrode
in saturated KCl solution
with semi-permeable
membrane

2. WHAT ARE THE SOURCES OF ELECTRICAL INTERFERENCE IN BIOLOGICAL SIGNALS?

> ⊃ Electrical interference is either due to external causes or to the patient. The former is most commonly due to the AC mains current, and the latter due to skeletal muscle action potentials either due to movement or shivering.

Mains current interference may occur if there is capacitive coupling between the mains and the patient. If a live conductor is close to the patient (not necessarily touching) then that lead tends to act as one plate of a capacitor, with the patient as the other plate. The circuit is completed because both are connected to earth. As the current in the live lead alternates between positive and negative the charge on the other side of the capacitor alternates similarly. This can be picked up on recording electrodes (e.g. the ECG) and is seen as a 50 Hz signal on the recording. This can be reduced either by moving the patient away from the live conductor, or by providing an earthed screen between the two 'plates' of the capacitor. This then discharges the charge from the live plate to earth and reduces the effect. Screened electrode leads consist of a wire mesh around the electrode that is connected to earth. A further cause of mains interference is by the interaction between the patient as a conductor in the changing magnetic field generated by the electromagnetic effect of the live conductor.

The most effective way to remove these signals is to have a 'common' lead in the ECG equipment that allows subtraction of those parts of the signal that are common to all the electrodes – called **common mode rejection**.

Patient interference is due to the presence of other electrical activity that is being measured. Anything that increases the amplitude of these signals, or reduces the amplitude of the signal being measured, will increase the effect of this interference. The most common problem is due to skeletal muscle activity especially during shivering, and everything should be done to ensure that the measured signal is maximised (by reducing the resistance at the patient connection) and that activity is minimised by keeping the patient warm and asking them to stop moving.

---

3. WHAT METHODS ARE AVAILABLE TO MEASURE CO_2 IN GASES?

⊃ **The method seen most frequently in anaesthetic practice uses absorption of infrared light.**

For measurement methods to be of use to anaesthetists they must be:

- Accurate to clinical levels
- Repeatable
- Easy and relatively quick to calibrate, and allow quick re-calibration if there is drift in the calibration
- Have a short response time so breath-to-breath measurements can be taken and the shape of the waveform displayed
- Able to measure other respiratory gases of interest particularly inhalational anaesthetic agent levels
- Not be significantly affected by the presence of other gases or water vapour

There are two methods seen in anaesthetic practice and other methods that may be of value in a research setting or in specific situations.

Practical methods that are seen in theatre use:

- **Infrared absorption** – A gas will absorb infrared (IR) radiation (wavelength $1 - 40$ μm), causing it to vibrate if it consists of more than one atom, and if those atoms are of different elements; so CO_2, N_2O, H_2O and volatile agents will absorb IR, while O_2 will not. The IR wavelength absorbed depends on the species (maximal at 4.26 μm for CO_2), and this allows IR absorption to identify different gases, the amount of light absorbed being in proportion to the amount of gas present. If the absorption at specific wavelengths is then compared with that of a reference gas, the concentration of CO_2 (and in some cases other gases) may be measured. Modern infrared analysers display concentrations of many respiratory gases (including carbon dioxide, nitrous oxide and volatile anaesthetic agents). However, errors may be seen due to interference by oxygen, which broadens the carbon dioxide spectra, and interference between gases (especially N_2O and CO_2 and carbon dioxide as the spectra overlap substantially). Water vapour also absorbs infrared light and this can cause falsely high readings. If the radiation is pulsed, sound is generated in proportion to the amount of gas present; this is the photoacoustic variation of spectroscopy.
- **Raman scattering** – In this method, gas is drawn from the breathing system and is exposed to monochromatic light from an argon laser. The energy from the light is absorbed by the intermolecular bonds and then is partially re-emitted at new wavelengths by the molecules. The wavelength shift and the scattering may be used to measure the concentration of the gases in the system. This technique allows measurement of all of the gases normally of interest in a breathing system (including CO_2, N_2O, O_2, N_2 and volatile anaesthetic agents). It is small and portable and the gases may be returned to the breathing system unchanged, however it does not have the

response rate suitable for paediatric monitoring (small tidal volumes and high respiratory rates).

Other Methods

- **Mass spectrometer –** Gas is drawn from the breathing system into the spectrometer where it is ionised then exposed to a magnetic field in a vacuum chamber. The various gases are separated according to their mass: charge ratio. The concentration of various gases of known mass: charge ratio may then be calculated. The spectrometer is highly accurate, reproducible and allows the measurement of many gases, however it is very bulky and expensive, and is susceptible to damage from water and some drugs. The gases cannot be returned to the breathing system, so they should be scavenged.

- **Calorimetric measurement –** If CO_2 is hydrated, the result is carbonic acid, which can therefore be measured by pH-sensitive means (e.g. using colour change). Detectors that use this principle are small and portable but only give a crude assessment of CO_2 level (low, normal, high).

---

4. WHAT IS A CAPNOGRAPH?

> ⊃ **The capnograph is regarded by many as the single most useful monitor in theatre.**

A capnograph is a device that **records** and shows a **graphical display** of CO_2 concentration. It produces a capnogram, which is a graphical plot of CO_2 against time. A capnometer is an instrument for measuring the numerical concentration of CO_2. Thus, all capnographs are capnometers, but a capnometer does not display a capnogram.

A real-time capnogram waveform displays a trace at 12.5 mm/sec, demonstrating fine detail and sudden changes in morphology. A trend capnogram waveform displays at 25 mm/min, demonstrating gradual changes over time. The delay time is the sum of the transit time and the rise time, where the transit time is the time taken for a sample to be delivered from the point of interest to the analyser, and the rise time is the time taken by the capnographic cell to register from 10% to 90% of a step change after the sample has entered the measuring chamber. The latter is also known as the response time, and is important, as it must be less than the time taken for one breath.

There are two common structural arrangements of capnographs – mainstream and sidestream.

Mainstream is an arrangement where the analysing cell is interposed in the breathing system. This type does not cause turbulent flow in the breathing system nor does it extract much gas from it (both of importance in paediatric anaesthesia). It also has a short delay time, but is vulnerable to being dropped and damaged. Mainstream devices are also heavy and difficult to support when using a mask. They can become hot and could burn patients.

Sidestream analysis requires a continuous sample to be drawn at the rate of (usually) 150 ml/min from the breathing system and analysed within the machine. This is a more common arrangement than mainstream, but the gas needs to be scavenged, or returned to the system if a circle is in use. Condensation forms and a water-trap is needed. It has a slower response time and is prone to diffusion errors and occlusion, however, its construction allows all the expensive parts of the system to be protected within a strong box which is important for prolonged reliability in a busy theatre environment.

Both types require calibration before and at intervals during use against room air (presumed to have zero CO_2) and an occasional calibration against a standard gas mixture.

---

5. WHAT PATTERNS MAY BE SEEN ON THE CAPNOGRAM AND WHAT DO THEY REPRESENT?

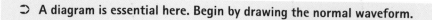

⊃ A diagram is essential here. Begin by drawing the normal waveform.

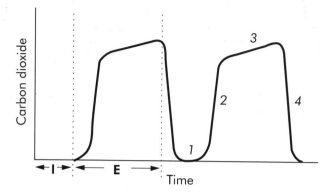

I = inspiration, E = expiration.

The phases of the normal waveform are as follows.

1: Inspiration: should be at zero, since any elevation of the baseline indicates rebreathing which may be seen with the Mapleson D arrangement.
2: Upslope phase. If this is shallow, this indicates obstruction.
3: Plateau. This represents mixing of alveolar gas, and if sloped rather than flat, indicates uneven mixing, as in chronic airways disease.
4: Fall to zero at start of inspiration.

These are some abnormal patterns:

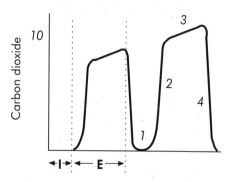

Malignant hyperpyrexia:
High plateau PCO_2, rapid rate.

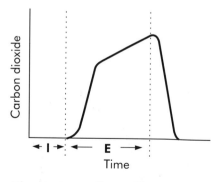

Chronic airways disease: Slow upstroke, wide $P(a\text{-}ET)CO_2$ gradient.

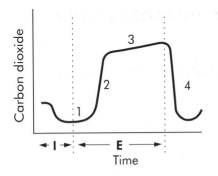

Defective valves in a circle system:
Raised baseline with oscillations.

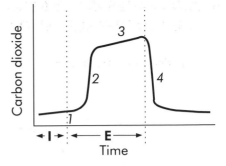

CO_2 rebreathing: Raised baseline.

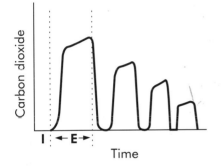

Reduced cardiac output: Progressive
diminution in amplitude.

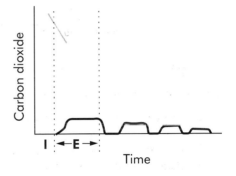

Oesophageal intubation: Even with
carbonated drink in stomach, less than 6
deflections will be seen. Thereafter, the
tube cannot be in the trachea if no CO_2 is
detected, unless circulatory arrest has
occurred.

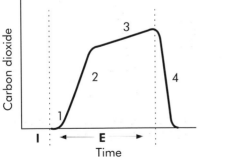

Airway obstruction: Slow ascent phase 2.

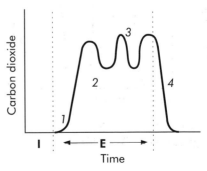

Recovery from neuromuscular blockade
during positive pressure ventilation: Clefts
are seen during phase 3.

6. HOW MAY TEMPERATURE BE MEASURED?

> ⊃ **Temperature is a measure of the tendency of an object to gain or lose heat in contact with another object of different temperature. It is not a measure of the heat content or molecular excitation of an object.**

The techniques for measuring temperature are based on this definition of temperature, as heat will travel from a warmer object to a colder one until the temperature difference is eliminated.

The oldest form of thermometer, as well as the most widely used, is the **mercury-in-glass thermometer**. This relies on the principle that the mercury receives heat from the object and that its volume changes in proportion to that temperature change. It is effective in the range –39°C to ~250°C. If a thermometer is required for lower temperatures, the **alcohol-in-glass thermometer** can be used (utilising the same principles) in the range –117°C to 78°C.

A wider range can be obtained by using gas thermometers, which use the principles of the gas laws. The volume of a gas at fixed pressure (or the pressure of gas at fixed volume) alter proportionally to the change in temperature. Although inconvenient to use, they have an effective range of –269°C to ~1600°C. They are generally used for the calibration of other thermometers.

The Platinum Resistance Thermometer measures the change in electrical resistance of a length of pure platinum wire with change in temperature. The resistance increases with increasing temperature, but the change is not linear so calibration is required against a gas thermometer. It has a wide range (-250°C to ~1300°C). The resistance is then measured using a Wheatstone bridge.

The thermistor is convenient for use in theatres. It is a semi-conductor device that has a reducing resistance with increasing temperature. Although the change is non-linear, it can be manufactured so that over the working range (body temperature plus or minus 25°C) it is *almost* linear. Thermistors can also be made small enough to be both fast responding and convenient for clinical use. They do, however, tend to alter their characteristics over time ('drift') or if subjected to high temperatures (e.g. in an autoclave) so they need to be recalibrated from time to time.

Another device seen in the laboratory is the **thermocouple**. This depends on the 'Seebeck effect'. When two conductors of different metals are connected together, a potential difference is generated that is directly related to the temperature at the junction. If the circuit is the completed by another junction (the reference junction), the current produced is non-linearly related to the temperature difference between the two junctions. Thus, if the temperature of the reference junction is known, the temperature of the measurement junction can be measured. The measurement junction can be made very small and so have a very fast response and may be made in the form of a needle.

---

7. HOW DOES A CLARK ELECTRODE WORK?

⊃ **The Clark electrode is a polarographic electrode for measurement of the oxygen tension within a gas or liquid.**

A Clark electrode (named after its inventor Leland Clark) actually consists of two electrodes – a platinum cathode and a silver/silver chloride anode. These are linked by a electrolyte medium containing potassium chloride. If a voltage (0.6V) is applied across the two electrodes the current that flows is proportional to the concentration of oxygen present, and thus this can be measured.

At the cathode, each oxygen atom combines with four electrons to form four hydroxyl ions:

$$O_2 + 4e^- + 2H_2O \Rightarrow 4OH^-$$

As the oxygen supply is rate-limiting the rate of reaction is proportional to it, and this is dependant on oxygen tension at the cathode. Hence the current flow is proportional to the oxygen tension.

The potassium chloride electrolytic medium is separated from the sample by a plastic membrane, and the oxygen tension equilibrates across the membrane. The electrode needs to be maintained at body temperature in order to make the results relevant.

The membrane may become coated with protein deposits or damaged and this can lead to inaccuracies.

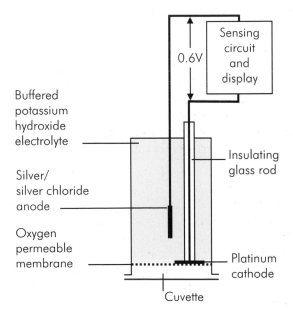

8. WHAT IS AN ISOBESTIC POINT?

⊃ In any mixture of two gases a point at which the absorption coefficients
  are identical is called an isobestic point. The most important one in
  anaesthetic practice is at 805 nm seen in a mixture of the oxygenated
  and deoxygenated forms of haemoglobin, which forms one of the points
  used in the algorithm of the pulse oximeter cicuitry.

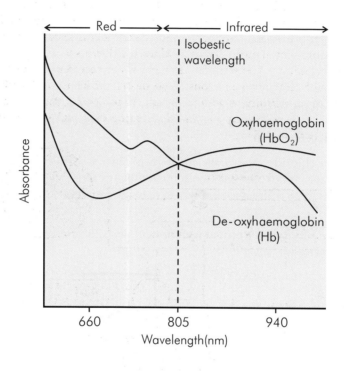

9. HOW DOES THE OSCILLOTONOMETER WORK?

⊃ **The oscillotonometer uses two cuffs, one to occlude arterial pulsations and one to sense pulsations and amplify them by a sensitive aneroid chamber.**

The oscillotonometer (eponymously known as von Recklinghausen's oscillotonometer) consists of a double cuff, an inflating bulb, two separate aneroid capsules within a sealed unit, a lever and a dial. The upper (proximal) cuff is the occluding cuff and is 5 cm wide, the lower (distal) is the sensing cuff and is 10 cm wide. The two cuffs overlap. The coarse aneroid chamber is sealed and responds to changes in pressure within the sealed case, which it transmits to a gauge by means of a rack and pinion device. The sensitive chamber is connected to the distal, sensing cuff. The lever operates in two positions. In position 1, which is the default position, the inflating bulb communicates with both cuffs. In position 2, there is a communication between the sensitive capsule and the sensing cuff, and the pressure relief valve allows the cuffs to deflate.

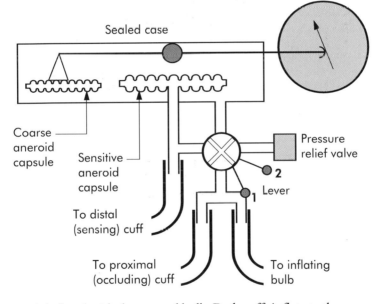

The system is inflated with the manual bulb. Both cuffs inflate to the same pressure, which is in continuity with the inside of the sealed case. The coarse chamber is compressed and the pressure indicated on the gauge, since a rack and pinion device connects the two. Once inflated above systolic, the lever is moved to position 2. As the occluding cuff deflates, pulsations will reach the sensing cuff and fluctuations will occur in the sensitive capsule. The fluctuations distort the sensitive chamber, changing the pressure within the sealed case. These pulsations are transmitted to the gauge. Oscillations will appear at systolic pressure, become maximal at mean arterial pressure, and disappear at diastolic pressure.

10. HOW DOES A PULSE OXIMETER WORK AND WHAT ARE THE PROBLEMS ASSOCIATED WITH ITS USE?

> ⊃ The pulse oximeter relies on measurement of the different absorption of oxyhaemoglobin and deoxyhaemoglobin at two different wavelengths.

The oximeter emits pulses of infrared (940 nm) and red (660 nm) light from two distinct LED's every 5 – 10 μsec. It then aims to identify the points of maximum (systole) and minimum (diastole) absorption. It measures the pulsatile component of the absorption at each of the two wavelengths and subtracts the constant component (i.e. that part that is not due to arterial blood). It then compares the absorption at the two different wavelengths and compares the ratio to an algorithm calculated from experimental data. The oxygenated haemoglobin absorbs more infrared light and less red light than the deoxygenated molecule. Pulse oximetry is most accurate above 90% oxyhaemoglobin saturation, and much less accurate below 80%. The machines are calibrated against healthy volunteers, which makes calibration to values below 85% ethically unacceptable.

Errors in calculating the pulsatile component of the light absorption

- *Failure due to low pulse pressure, vasoconstriction, hypotension and venous pulsation*
  All of these make it harder for the oximeter to define the points of maximum and minimum absorption (systole and diastole).

- *Interference* from abnormal haemoglobins (e.g. carboxyhaemoglobin or methaemoglobin) or intravenous compounds or dyes (e.g. bilirubin, methylene blue, indocyanine green).

These will all affect the pulsatile component and so are entered in the machine's calculation of the saturation. The functional saturation (ratio of oxygenated haemoglobin to haemoglobin that is available for oxygenation) is therefore altered. Bilirubin absorption is similar to that of deoxygenated haemoglobin and so gives a falsely low reading for HbO. Carboxyhaemoglobin, which has an absorption is similar to oxyhaemoglobin, will give a misleadingly high reading for HbO. Methaemoglobin, which has an absorption that is similar at the two wavelengths monitored, tends to produce a SpO_2 that approaches 85%. Foetal haemoglobin has no effect.

- *Irregular pulse rate*
  Atrial fibrillation and other arrhythmias make it harder for the machine to predict the points of maximum and minimum absorption.

Increase of the ratio of the non-pulsatile component of the light absorption

- *Nail varnish and dirt or staining on fingers*
  These tend to increase the non-pulsatile absorption and so will make the pulsatile component relatively small and less sensitive.

- *Optical interference*
  Light from room lights, especially if it is flickering (and so 'pulsatile') can

affect the SpO_2. Normally, in excess ambient light, the oximeter will fail to provide a reading, and the probe should be shielded.

Machine dysfunction

Electrical interference

Diathermy will affect the reading circuitry in the oximeter and this normally causes loss of the reading, and occasionally inaccurate pulse rates.

Other problems related to the physiology of oxygen saturation

Saturation is of little value in assessing high oxygen tensions

Because of the shape of the haemoglobin dissociation curve the oximeter is unable to differentiate high but safe oxygen tensions from those that may be excessive and risk toxicity.

Oximetry is a poor monitor of ventilatory or airway failure

Arterial oxygenation is a late indicator of hypoventilation or failure of the airway (e.g. oesophageal intubation) and must not be relied on as a monitor of this.

Finally it should be noted that oximeters may be a danger to the patient.

- There are a number of reports of pressure damage especially in those patients monitored for prolonged periods with low peripheral perfusion pressures.
- A number of patients have suffered burns from the probe, either due to incompatibility in probe and monitor or when some oximeters are used in MRI scanners.

---

11. HOW CAN YOU MEASURE BLOOD PRESSURE?

⊃ **Blood pressure can be measured invasively, which involves cannulating an artery, or non-invasively.**

Invasive blood pressure monitoring

This may be performed at any accessible peripheral artery, the radial being the most popular. The risk to vessel patency increases with the duration of cannulation. A 20G teflon cannula is used. The other requirements are:

1. A column of fluid in a short (less than 120 cm), wide-bore (1.5 – 3.0 mm internal diameter), rigid tube free from air. If the tubing is too long, resonance will occur; if compliant, or if air is in the system, there will be excessive damping of the signal.
2. A pressure transducer. This converts energy in one form (pressure), into another (electricity).
3. Amplifier and signal-processor.
4. Display. This may be on a cathode ray tube, or on a digital readout, or commonly both. The advantage of the latter arrangement is that accurate numerical data is combined with a visual impression of the waveform, allowing other information to be derived from it.

The advantages of invasive monitoring are:

1. Continuous information, on a beat-to-beat basis. Non-invasive blood pressure (NIBP) measurement can be repeated only up to once a minute, as this is the interval the machine requires to take the measurement.
2. Continuous measurement is more accurate.
3. Other information can be derived from the signal:
   - Heart rate
   - Stroke volume, from the area under the curve
   - Contractility, from the gradient of the up-slope
   - Resistance and compliance of the arterial tree, from the diastolic delay
   - Myocardial work and O_2 consumption, which is proportional to the area under the curve of systolic pressure and time
   - Myocardial perfusion, which is proportional to the area under the curve of diastolic pressure and time
   - The effect of any arrhythmia is immediately apparent from the amplitude of the pressure wave corresponding to the abnormal QRS complex
   - Patient-ventilator interaction. In ventilated patients variation in beat-to-beat systolic pressure (SPV) or pulse (systolic–diastolic) pressure (PPV) is highly correlated to that patient's response to fluid loading and is thus a measure of preload

Invasive monitoring of blood pressure was first performed by a clergyman, Stephen Hales in 1733, on a conscious horse, using a column of water.

Non-invasive blood pressure monitoring

This may be performed as follows:

1. Use of a Riva-Rocci cuff and auscultation of the Korotkoff sounds. See Question 21 (p59)
2. Use of an automated blood pressure machine
3. By an oscillotonometer

---

12. WHAT IS PARAMAGNETISM?

> ⊃ Paramagnetism is the property of a gas that is attracted to a magnetic field and is the opposite of diamagnetism, which is to be repelled by a magnetic field. It is a principle employed in oxygen analysis.

Oxygen (and nitric oxide) are paramagnetic whereas other gases tend to be diamagnetic. This is due to the configuration of the electrons in the outer shell of the molecules. A differential pressure transducer is suspended between the sample gas, containing oxygen of unknown concentration, and a reference gas, which is air, and has a known oxygen concentration.

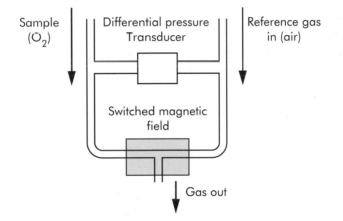

A strong, pulsed magnetic field is applied over the junction of the two gases. There will then be a correspondingly pulsed pressure change between the two tubes if there is a difference in the oxygen concentration, and hence the paramagnetic tendency, of the two samples. The pressure difference can then be calibrated against different oxygen concentrations.

13. WHAT IS THE PIEZO-ELECTRIC EFFECT?

⊃ **The piezo-electric effect is the property of a substance such that it generates an electric charge when exposed to pressure.**

This effect implies the presence of a transducer, and is the basis of ultrasound. Ultrasound is generated by employing the piezo-electric effect in reverse: in other words, a high frequency voltage is applied to a crystal that then oscillates at the frequency of the applied potential difference, generating ultrasound radiation. The ultrasound transducer performs two tasks; it generates and transmits ultrasound radiation, and it also senses the returned signal. The returned ultrasound signal is again transduced into electrical energy and displayed as an image.

⊃ **This may be linked to a question on ultrasound and its use.**

14. HOW DOES ULTRASOUND WORK?

⊃ **Ultrasound detects soft tissue interfaces by the reflection of ultrasound radiation.**

Waves in water oscillate at right angles to the direction of travel of the wave. Sound waves by contrast are transmitted by oscillation of particles in the direction of propagation of the wave.

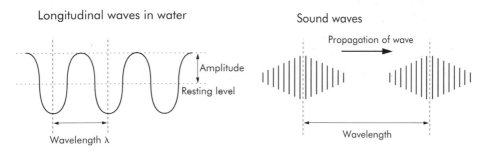

The speed at which the wave moves $= \lambda f$ where the wavelength is denoted by λ, and the frequency by f, which determines the pitch of the sound. The amplitude of the wave determines the loudness. Ultrasound is sound whose pitch (i.e. frequency) is above that audible to the human ear – above 20,000 Hz, although clinical ultrasound operates between 1 and 10 MHz, some 50,000 times higher than the audible range.

Ultrasound is absorbed by tissues (attenuation) and reflected by tissue interfaces. The extent to which the signal is attenuated depends on the nature of the tissue and on the frequency of the radiation. Bone and air have the highest attenuation coefficients, and water the smallest; this is why ultrasound travels badly through air-filled cavities such as gut and lung, and why a full bladder is used as a 'window' for ultrasound imaging of the gravid uterus. There is a balance to be struck between penetration of tissues and resolution of images. The lowest frequency ultrasound achieves the highest tissue penetration, but low frequency implies long wavelength as the two are inversely related.

Long wavelength is associated with lower resolution. The solution is to use ultrasound of the highest frequency (and shortest wavelength, and best resolution) that will just penetrate tissue adequately. This in turn depends on the nature of the tissue, so 3–5 MHz is used for abdominal scanning and 10 MHz for the eye.

---

15. WHAT IS DOPPLER ULTRASOUND?

⊃ **In 1842, Christian Doppler (an Austrian physicist) discovered that the shift in the reflected frequency of an optic wave is proportional to the velocity at which the reflecting object is moving.**

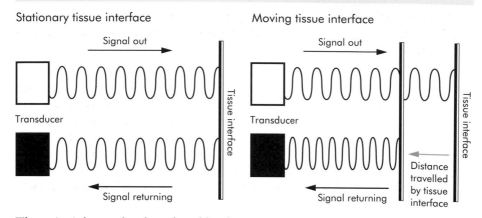

The principle can be thought of by first imagining the wave reflected off a still mirror and then measuring the frequency of the peaks of the waves as they hit the mirror, and then as they reach a receiver. Now if the mirror is moving towards the waves then the wave peaks will reach the mirror quicker and be reflected as a wave with the peaks closer together and so a higher frequency. This change can be displayed audibly or visually, using colour to indicate velocity. The wave used is of ultrasonic frequency, and the frequency is adjusted to change the depth at which measurements are made (high frequencies are for superficial measurements whereas lower frequencies allow deeper measurement).

Doppler ultrasound is used in adult echocardiography, in foetal echocardiography, and in the measurement of uterine artery flow. In vascular surgery it is used to confirm the patency of vessels. It may also be used to measure blood pressure by detection of vessel wall motion.

A Duplex scanner is one that combines real-time ultrasound with Doppler imaging.

The velocity of the blood is calculated by referring to the equation:

$$\text{Velocity} = \frac{\delta f \cdot V_{sound}}{2f \cdot \cos \theta}$$

where:
δf = Doppler shift in frequency

V_{sound} = Velocity of sound in tissue

f = Initial frequency of the ultrasound wave

θ = Incident angle of the beam to the blood movement. If this is less than 30% then $\cos \theta$ approximates to 1.

16. HOW DOES MAGNETIC RESONANCE IMAGING WORK?

> ⊃ Magnetic resonance imaging (MRI) depends on absorption of electromagnetic radiation by, and emission of radio frequency radiation from, atomic nuclei.

MRI was originally known as nuclear magnetic resonance (probably a better term). The word "nuclear" was removed to alleviate public concerns about ionising radiation, which does not feature in the technique.

Every proton in an atomic nucleus has a single positive charge. Protons act in pairs, each with opposite spin characteristics that cancel out. In an atom with an odd number of protons, (such as H^+, ^{13}C) one proton will be unpaired and will have spin and charge. Normally this is irrelevant, but if exposed to an electromagnetic field, the nucleus containing an unpaired proton will align itself along the axis of the magnetic field. When the electromagnetic field is withdrawn, the atomic nucleus reverts to its original position, and in so doing, releases energy as radio waves. The energy involved is very small, so MRI can only be used to detect substances present in at least millimolar concentrations.

MRI can be used to define anatomy in axial computed tomography, like the X-ray based equivalent, but with better views of the soft tissues and in particular the posterior fossa of the skull. MRI can also perform spectroscopic analysis of biochemical processes.

T_1 and T_2 refer to the relaxation time constants, where T_2 is the spin-spin relaxation constant, the time taken for the decay of the signal. T_1 is the spin-lattice relaxation time.

Magnetic field strengths

The magnetic field strengths used in MRI are considerable. The earth's magnetic field is of the order of 1 Gauss; 1 tesla (1 T) = 10,000 Gauss. The fields in MRI scanners are between 0.05 and 2.0 tesla. Around the machine there will be a measurable fringe field, within which ferromagnetic items (bleeps, needles, stethoscopes, gas cylinders) may be subjected to movement but which will also distort the image generated by the machine. The fringe field may be defined in terms of the 50 Gauss and 5 Gauss lines; these lie about 8 m from the machine, or less depending on the shielding on the equipment.

---

17. WHAT ARE THE PROBLEMS WHEN PERFORMING ANAESTHESIA FOR MRI SCANNING?

⊃ **This concerns the enclosed space of an MRI scanner (smaller space than a conventional CT) and the exposure to the powerful electromagnetic field.**

▨ Sedation is often required because the MRI environment is extremely claustrophobic and noisy. Children and anxious adults may need to be anaesthetised for scanning to take place, which may take up to an hour – this is longer than for a conventional CT.

▨ Access to the anaesthetised patient is a concern because of the enclosed space and because of the delay in extracting the patient from the machine should it become necessary.

▨ Regarding the effects of the magnetic field:
   ▨ Ferromagnetic objects will be subjected to force sufficient to move them in fields over 50 Gauss, and so must be placed outside the marked 50 Gauss line.
   ▨ Infusion devices fail in fields over 100 Gauss.
   ▨ Pacemakers fail in fields over 5 Gauss.
   ▨ Electric cable may have a current induced within it by the magnet and heat up as a consequence. Cabling must be minimised and where present, insulated.

⊃ **In anaesthesia for CT, the anaesthetic machine and the monitoring can be there, but the anaesthetist cannot; in anaesthesia for MRI, the anaesthetist can be there but the equipment cannot.**

▨ *Induction*: Conventional, performed outside the magnetic field.

▨ *Airway*: RAE polar tracheal tube, which contours snugly around the face and connects to a breathing system, which should be a coaxial arrangement at least 10 m long.

▨ *Maintenance*: Spontaneous respiration or IPPV with the anaesthetic machine outside the 50 Gauss line. There are nonmagnetic anaesthetic machines available, which include aluminium cylinders. Volatiles and total intravenous techniques have both been used.

▨ *Monitoring*: The dorsalis pedis pulse may be accessible. An oesophageal stethoscope is useful. Capnography with extended tubing is possible, but the delay time is extended. Non-ferromagnetic ECG electrodes should be used.

▨ *Reversal*: Remove the patient from the field before allowing them to wake up.

---

18. HOW DO YOU MONITOR THE NEUROMUSCULAR JUNCTION?

> ⟳ You should describe a typical nerve stimulator. This delivers 50 mA for
> 0.2 – 1.0 msec, and requires 50 – 300 V. It is applied over the course of
> a mixed peripheral nerve, which it then stimulates while the anaesthetist
> observes muscle function in the distribution of the nerve. The nerve
> stimulator is therefore a monitor of the neuromuscular junction.

Four tests are used to detect type of, degree of, reversibility of, and recovery from,
neuromuscular block.

Twitch-tetanus-twitch
This distinguishes the *type* of block; four patterns are observed.

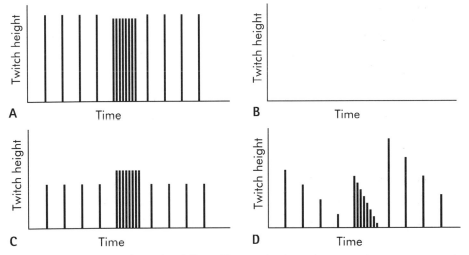

A: Normal – symmetrical twitches followed by sustained tetanic contraction; no post-tetanic
facilitation (PTF). **B**: Total block; no response. **C**: Partial depolarising block – weak but
symmetrical twitches; sustained contracture; no PTF. **D**: Partial non-depolarising block –
weak twitches, fade on tetanic stimulus, PTF.

Train of four
train of four consists of four identical stimuli delivered at 2 Hz. This distinguishes
the degree of block. It is possible to use the count, or the ratio of force of 4th to 1st
twitch (T_4: T_1).

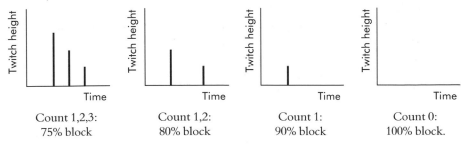

| Count 1,2,3: | Count 1,2: | Count 1: | Count 0: |
| 75% block | 80% block | 90% block | 100% block. |

Post-tetanic twitch count

This determines the *reversibility* of a non-depolarising block; the device delivers 50 Hz for 5 sec, then 1 Hz, counting detectable twitches. Reversal is possible if count is greater than 10.

Double burst

This uses a pair of bursts of 3 pulses at 50 Hz pulses separated by 0.75 sec. It assesses *recovery* from non-depolarising block, displaying the T_1: T_4 ratio.

_____

19. WHAT ARE THE CHARACTERISTIC COMPONENTS OF THE CVP TRACE AND WHAT AFFECTS THEM?

> ⊃ There are three waves (a, c and v) and two descents (x and y)

a wave
- This is produced by the contraction of the right atrium (atrial systole). It is therefore absent in atrial fibrillation. It is increased by anything that impedes right atrial emptying (tricuspid or pulmonary stenosis, right ventricular hypertrophy, pulmonary hypertension). Heart block leads to variable a waves, and complete heart block may lead to 'cannon' waves when the right atrial contracts against the closed tricuspid valve.

c wave
- This occurs just after the onset of ventricular systole and is caused by the leaflets of the tricuspid valve bulging into the right atrium during the initial isovolumetric ventricular contraction.

v wave
- This is caused by the filling of the right atrium against the closed tricuspid valve. In tricuspid incompetence it is increased by the back flow of blood from the right ventricle during ventricular systole and so will be very prominent.

x descent
- This is the result of the relaxation of the atrium and the downward movement of the tricuspid leaflets as the ventricle contracts during the ejection phase. It does not occur if the tricuspid valve is incompetent.

y descent
- This occurs when the tricuspid valve opens and blood flows from the right atrium to the right ventricle.
- After the **y descent** there is a small deflection in the ascending limb of the **a wave**, this is due to the completion of passive ventricular filling, is known as the **h wave**. This can normally only be seen in bradycardia.

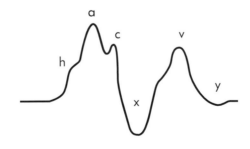

Normal CVP trace

20. HOW DO YOU MEASURE FUNCTIONAL RESIDUAL CAPACITY?

> ⊃ **Functional residual capacity (FRC) is the lung volume in which gas exchange takes place.**

A drawing or the spirometry is very useful, and demonstrates that you at least know what FRC represents.

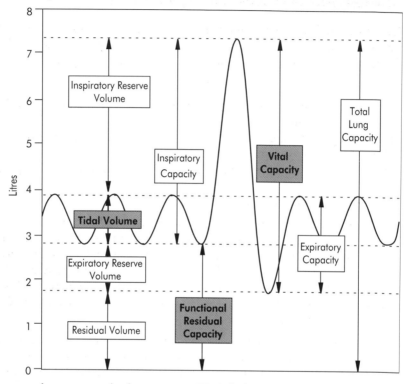

There are at least two methods to measure FRC, helium dilution and plethysmography.

Helium dilution:
This involves breathing an oxygen-enriched gas mixture with a known concentration of helium, from a circle system with a carbon dioxide absorber. Helium is not taken up by the circulation, and so if the volume of the apparatus is known, and the final concentration of helium is measured, this allows measurement of total lung capacity.

$$[He]_{Initial} \times Vol_{equip} = [He]_{equilibrium} \times Vol_{(equipment\ +\ total\ lung\ capacity)}$$

One can derive residual volume and FRC, by using spirometry and arithmetic. However, Helium dilution cannot measure that volume which is behind closed airways, because the helium cannot get there.

Body plethysmograph:
In order to measure FRC in, for example, a patient with emphysema and airway closure, the body plethysmograph must be used. This uses Boyle's law, $P1 \times V1 = P2 \times V2$.

21. WHAT IS THE PRINCIPLE BEHIND THE 'RIVA-ROCCI' CUFF AND KOROTKOFF SOUNDS AND HOW MAY THEY BE INACCURATE?

⊃ The Riva-Rocci cuff (named after an Italian doctor) was first described as a measurement of blood pressure one hundred years ago in 1896. Initially the systolic pressure was determined by palpation; Nikolai Korotkoff reported an auscultatory method in 1905.

The Riva-Rocci cuff is the eponymous name for the blood pressure cuff and the Korotkoff sounds are the noises heard over the brachial artery during deflation of an occluding proximal cuff and are taken as measurements of blood pressure.

Korotkoff originally described three sounds; five are now described.

Phase I: Appearance of a tapping sound, corresponding to the systolic pressure.

Phase II: Muffling or disappearance of sounds; "auscultatory gap".

Phase III: Sounds reappear.

Phase IV: Sounds become muffled again. This is taken as diastolic pressure in the UK.

Phase V: Sounds disappear.

Although there is no definite answer to what causes the sounds it seems reasonable to assume that the sounds are created by turbulent flow causing vibration of the arterial wall, and the sound is subsequently amplified and transmitted through the tissues to the stethoscope. When the pressure within the vessel changes as the systolic pulsation passes it reaches a point when the pressure difference across the vessel wall is zero. This is highly conductive to vessel wall vibration and so the vibrations are heard when the cuff pressure is between systolic and diastolic pressures.

There is some discussion as to whether Korotkoff phase IV (sudden muffling of the sounds) or phase V (disappearance of the sounds) should be used for the diastolic pressure. Both slightly over-read in comparison with direct methods (phase IV more so), but phase V is said to be a gradual process and so the exact point is difficult to determine, and in high output states (such as pregnancy) phase V may not occur until the cuff is fully deflated.

Errors in the reading of blood pressure relate to:

Cuff width – A narrow cuff will give an overly high reading and a wide cuff too low a reading. The cuff width is said to need to be 2/3rds of the length of the forearm.

Cuff length – The inflating part of the cuff must lie over the artery so that the pressure within the cuff is the same as the pressure that is transmitted to the vessel wall.

Aneroid gauges – Errors in the zeroing and calibration of these gauges are common causes of error in their use.

Atherosclerosis – The vessel walls tend to be stiffer and so the vibration is reduced, and its frequency may fall below the audible range, making the sounds dfficult to hear.

Hypotension – Sounds become much more difficult to hear.

22. HOW MAY CEREBRAL BLOOD FLOW BE MEASURED?

⊃ Mean cerebral blood flow is about 55 ml/100 g/min and is maintained within a relatively narrow range compared to other organs. It varies between the anatomical structures of the brain with grey matter in general receiving more than twice (70 ml/100 g/min) the blood flow of white matter (30 ml/100 g/min).

The brain consumes approximately 3.5 ml/100 g/min of oxygen leaving the jugular venous blood 65% saturated.

Cerebral blood flow can be estimated by:

- *Kety method* – An application of the Fick principle which determines the total cerebral blood flow in ml/100 g/min. Nitrous oxide is used as the transported substance because it has partition coefficient of 1, which ensures that the brain concentration becomes equal to the jugular venous concentration, after an equilibration time of 10 minutes. A subject breathes 15% nitrous oxide for 10 minutes. The total nitrous oxide transferred to 100 g of brain tissue per minute (Q) can be determined from the final nitrous oxide content of 100g of jugular venous blood divided by 10. The average arteriovenous difference (D) in nitrous oxide content per millilitre is determined from arterial and venous samples during equilibration. The blood flow can then be calculated from the ratio Q / D.
- *Scintillography* – Using radioactive tracers (xenon) to trace regional blood flow.
- *SPECT scanning* – Scintillography enhanced by CT or MRI scanning.
- *PET scanning* – Use of 2-deoxyglucose labelled with a positron emitter.
- *Transcranial Doppler* – Crude but readily available for clinical use in ICU or operating theatre.

---

23. WHAT DEVICES MAY BE USED TO MEASURE TEMPERATURE?

⊃ **These may be classified as direct reading, where the display and site of measurement are in contact or remote reading where the display is remote from the measurement site.**

The choice of thermometer is determined by the application, the clinical environment, the required accuracy, and need for a continuous display.

Clinical measurement of temperature uses the following devices:

- Mercury glass thermometer
- Chemical thermometer
- Resistance thermometer
- Thermistors
- Thermocouples

(See Q 6 p 42)

Environmental temperature is usually measured by dial thermometers.

A note on Temperature scales:

- Fahrenheit (1714) developed this temperature scale using the first mercury thermometer. The zero point was set using a mixture of sodium chloride and ice. According to this scale, ice melted at 32°F, water boiled at 212°F, and body temperature was assumed to be 100°F.
- Centigrade (1742) is a scale developed by Celsius, having two fixed points, 0°C for the melting point of ice, and 100°C for the boiling point of water.
- Kelvin (absolute Temperature scale). This scale uses the absolute zero, recorded at the triple point of water –273.15°K. The boiling point of water according to this scale is 373.15°K.

24. WHAT IS THE DIFFERENCE BETWEEN ABSOLUTE AND RELATIVE HUMIDITY?

Absolute humidity is the mass of water vapour present in a given volume of gas at defined temperature and pressure (expressed as g of H_2O/m^3 of gas).

Relative humidity is the mass of water vapour present in a given volume of gas, expressed as a percentage of the mass of water vapour required to saturate the same volume of gas at identical temperature and pressure.

⊃ Note particularly that the amount of water vapour required to saturate a known volume of gas increases with temperature, i.e. a gas saturated at room temperature (20°C) contains less water than the same volume, saturated at body temperature (37°C).

From its definition, relative humidity (RH), can be calculated from the ratio of the mass of water vapour present (m_P), to the mass required for satruation (m_S) as follows:

$$RH \ = \ \frac{m_P}{m_S}$$

However from the gas laws, mass of a gas in a mixture is proportional to the partial pressure it exerts, thus:

$$RH \ = \ \frac{\text{water vapour pressure}}{\text{saturated water vapour pressure}}$$

Instruments used to measure humidity are called hygrometers. Examples include:

- Regnault's hygrometer
- Hair hygrometer
- Wet and dry bulb thermometers
- Humidity transducers

———————————————

25. CAN YOU QUANTIFY SOME COMMON BIOLOGICAL SIGNALS?

⊃ This question requires an answer explaining the voltage and frequency of EEG, ECG and EMG signals. The line of questioning will usually move on to the equipment needed to record these signals, often focussing on the characteristics of amplifiers.

COMMON BIOLOGICAL SIGNALS

Signal	Voltage range	Frequency range (Hz)
Electro-encephalogram (EEG)	1–500 μV	0–60
Electrocardiogram (ECG)	0.1–50 mV	0–100
Electromyogram (EMG)	0.01–100 mV	0–1000

3

QUESTIONS ON SAFETY

1. HOW DOES ELECTRICITY CAUSE MORBIDITY AND MORTALITY?

Consider classfying this topic in the following way:

- Electrocution
- Microshock
- Burns
- Ignition of flammable materials causing fires and explosions

⟳ **What mechanisms are there for electrical safety in the operating theatre?**

Mains supply

Isolation transformers
- Isolating transformers can supply all outlets of a theatre suite
- Problems if several pieces of equipment used that each have small leakage currents that sum up to enough to cut off the power
- Faults in one equipment may disrupt power to other equipment
- Isolation transformers can be used in individual pieces of equipment

Leakage current monitors
- Line isolation monitors measure potential for current flow from isolated power supply to ground. If too high, current flows to ground, alarm goes off or circuit breaks. Sensitive to a few milliamperes

Residual current circuit breakers
- Measures any imbalances of current in Neutral and Live lines
- Measures difference in magnetic flux between these two lines
- Breaks circuit if imbalance occurs

Earth Leakage Circuit Breaker
- Measures current in Earth line, should be zero. Disrupts circuit or sounds an alarm
- Not of use for Class 2 equipment as these are not earthed (see below)
- Differences of as little as 30 mA can trip the ELCB in milliseconds

Patient
- Isolated from earth

■ Electrical isolation of components in direct contact with the patient is achieved using isolating transformers, battery powered equipment that is isolated from earth or electro-optical links
■ Not touching metal conductors
■ Avoid low impedance earth connections
■ Avoid earth loops
■ Ensure good contact between neutral plate of diathermy and patient
■ Isolating capacitors in diathermy that have a high impedance to mains frequency (50 Hz) and low impedance to diathermy frequency (1 MHz)

2. DESCRIBE THE MAIN TYPES OF ELECTRICAL EQUIPMENT

⊃ Types of equipment: Class 1, 2 and 3 or Types B, BF, CF

Class 1 equipment
■ All accessible parts of this equipment are earthed
■ If a fault occurs that causes the casing to become "live" then a fuse blows and the life potential is removed from the case

Class 2 equipment
■ This not earthed but doubly insulated equipment
■ There is no possibility that a person will touch a conducting part

Class 3 equipment
■ No potentials greater than 24 V AC or 50 V DC
■ There is still a danger of microshock. as leakage currents may flow to electrical earth if insulation of "live" circuits deteriorate

The following classifications are based on maximum permissible leakage currents.

Type B
■ Can be from Class 1, 2 or 3 but maximum leakage current does not exceed 100 microamperes
■ This is not suitable for direct connection to the heart
■ Risk of microshock

Type BF
■ All patient circuits are electrically isolated from other parts of equipment
■ Maximum leakage current is also 100 microamperes
■ Not suitable for connection to the heart

Type CF
■ Maximum leakage current is less than 10 microamperes
■ Suitable for indirect cardiac connection (examples include ECG leads and thermodilution catheters)

Also: **No mobile phones in theatre because medical electronic equipment can behave like radio receivers and a mobile phone frequency signal could interfere with electronic equipment. Recommended exclusion zones – 10 metres maximum.**

3. WHAT ARE THE EFFECTS OF CURRENT AT 50 Hz?

10 μA	Absolute safety value for cardiac connections
100 μA	Can cause microshock; VF if directly connected to heart.
1 mA	Threshold of feeling
5 mA	Maximum safe current
8 mA	Burns
15 mA	"Let go" current limit; Victim is unable to "let go" due to tonic contraction of the flexor muscles
50 mA	Severe pain; Possible respiratory arrest
>100 mA	Ventricular fibrillation

---

4. WHAT FACTORS INCREASE THE CHANCES OF VENTRICULAR FIBRILLATION WITH ELECTRICAL EQUIPMENT?

Skin impedance
Impedance is greatest when skin is dry. Wet skin has low impedance and encourages current flow

Timing of shock in relation to ECG
Effective Refractory Period of cardiac muscle is 200 msec. If shock occurs during T wave (repolarisation of ventricles) then VF is more likely.

Sites of entry and exit
Maximum effect on the heart is seen with the greatest current density passing through the heart. Therefore, a current passing between the patient's arms has greater effect than one passing through the feet.

NB
- AC is worse than DC
- It takes 500 mA of DC to produce VF
- Patient may be predisposed to ventricular arrythmias

---

5. HOW CAN A PATIENT'S TEMPERATURE BE MAINTAINED DURING THE COURSE OF A LONG OPERATION?

⊃ The human is a homeotherm, with enzymatic, cerebral and muscular activity all depending on body temperature staying within the limits of 34–42°C. Postoperative hypothermia has particular implications for recovery of neuromuscular function.

Consider *attenuation of losses*, and *provision of heat*, separately.

Attenuation of heat loss

Loss occurs by means of radiation, convection, conduction and evaporation. The head is a particular source of radiant loss, especially in the neonate. Loss through convection is increased under anaesthesia because of vasodilation, and when body cavities are open, as at laparotomy. Radiant heat loss may be reduced by the use of a reflective "space blanket" while convective loss is minimised by keeping the patient covered. Conductive loss is less of a problem, other than in the case of administration of large amounts of cold fluid, which is to be avoided, use a fluid warmer. Evaporative loss from body cavities and expired gases is significant, and may be reduced by the use of heat and moisture exchangers (HME) and circle breathing systems.

The isothermic saturation boundary (ISB) is the point at which gas in the bronchial tree reaches 37°C and 100% humidity; this is normally at the carina. Breathing a dry gas mixture moves the ISB downwards, so that large airways are exposed to dry gases and so participate in heat and moisture exchange. One observed effect of an HME is to restore the ISB towards the normal position.

Active heating

Heat is generated by basal metabolism, which is reduced by anaesthesia, and by muscular activity, which is all but abolished when muscle relaxation is employed: not only are all muscles inactive, but there is no work of breathing as the patient's lungs are artificially ventilated.

Means of providing active warming include:

- Maintaining ambient temperature in theatre above 22°C
- Warming administered intravenous fluids
- Warming blankets on operating table
- Warming blanket in patient bed prior to transfer from operating table

6. WHAT DEVICES IN THE ANAESTHETIC MACHINE PREVENT BAROTRAUMA?

> ⊃ The supply for machines in theatre is by pipeline, with cylinders as back-up. The gases are delivered at 4 Bar (420 kPa, 60 psi).

Oxygen is stored in a Vacuum Insulated Evaporator (VIE) at –183°C and nitrous oxide is stored in a manifold of cylinders. After heat exchanging and pressure reduction, gases enter the theatre at terminal outlets, where a Schrader probe leads to a gas-specific hose, which in turn connects to a Non-Interchangeable Screw Thread (NIST) at the anaesthetic machine. There are either one or two pressure regulators (also called pressure reducing valves) within the machine (the number depends on the manufacturer) after which there is a pressure relief valve which operates at 800 kPa (8 Bar, 120 psi) in order to protect the machine (rather than the patient) from damage. On the back bar, where the vaporisers are situated, there is a pressure relief valve, which operates at 42 kPa (60 psi); it is this which protects the patient. The reservoir bag will also burst at less than one atmosphere.

---

7. WHAT FEATURES AND CONDUCT ARE IMPORTANT IN THE SAFE USE OF GAS CYLINDERS?

⊃ **These may be divided into storage, identification, testing and connection.**

Storage

A   Large cylinders should be stored upright, whilst smaller ones and importantly Entonox must be stored horizontally.

B   Cylinders should be kept indoors and protected from weather and extremes of temperature.

C   By using the cylinders in rotation the use of each cylinder is similar to that of all the others. This ensures that the interval between testing is appropriate.

D   Medical gases are stored separately from other gases and in the past when flammable gases were used these were stored separately from other medical gases.

E   The cylinders are made of manganese steel, high carbon steel or aluminium alloy to ensure that they are able to resist the high internal pressures. (Cylinders should be able to withstand approximately 170% of their maximum working pressure). It should be noted that even these materials do not stop the risk of explosion if the cylinder is dropped on a hard surface.

Identification

A   Cylinders may be identified by their colour coding and the system used in the UK is the international standard of colours for medical gases (ISO/R32). It should be noted that this standard despite being international is NOT worldwide (e.g. oxygen cylinders in the UK are black with white shoulders, but in the USA they are green and in Germany blue with white shoulders).

B   They are stamped with the owners mark (normally the gas supply company), a serial number, the testing pressure as well as a mark that records the pressure testing. They are also stamped with a safe filling pressure.

C   Cylinders also have clearly written labels permanently attached. This also contains information on the safety precautions required for use (particularly the avoidance of oil on cylinders of gases that support combustion (oxygen, Entonox and nitrous oxide).

Testing

A   Medical cylinders are regularly inspected and tested by the manufacturers, including endoscopic internal examination. Also one of each batch is tested to destruction during manufacture so the quality of the metal used for manufacture is ensured. Faulty cylinders are destroyed.

B   Cylinders in the UK have a plastic disc inserted between the valve and the body, the colour and shape of which is determined by the date of the last examination.

Connection

A   The cylinders that we use in theatre have a pin-index system on their valve bodies to ensure that accidental connection to the wrong yoke cannot occur.

B   Before attaching a new cylinder it is advisable to open the cylinder momentarily to blow out any dust that is lodged in the outlet of the cylinder to stop this entering the anaesthetic machine.

C   The cylinder should be turned on slowly to reduce the risk of adiabatic heating due to a rapid increase in pressure within the machine. The cylinder should be turned on fully to reduce the fall of pressure as the cylinder empties. When turning off the cylinder this should be done with only moderate force in order minimise damage to the valve seating.

---

8. WHY IS A PATIENT NOT ELECTROCUTED BY DIATHERMY?

The effects of an alternating current on tissues is related to the current density (current per unit area). High currents are focused onto small areas to cause the local burning that is the object of diathermy. However in order to be of a threat to the patient (not by burning him) the current must depolarise excitable tissue (nerves and muscle). It is this excitation of tissue that causes ventricular fibrillation. The susceptibility of the tissue to current is related to the frequency applied. If the frequency is between 40 and 60 Hz then the required current for ventricular fibrillation is small, and if applied directly to the heart is very small indeed (approximately 150 μA), however as the frequency is increased tissue becomes less and less susceptible to excitation, and at the frequencies used for diathermy (1 to 1.5 MHz) there is little muscle excitation even at currents high enough to cause burning.

---

9. WHAT IS THE STOICHIOMETRIC CONCENTRATION AND THE FLAMMABILITY LIMIT OF A MIXTURE?

> ⊃ The stoichiometric concentration is that relative concentration of the mixture of combustible agent (as vapour) and oxidising agent at which the reaction that occurs uses up all the available agents.

It is the concentration that the most complete reaction can happen for a given volume of combustible agent, and so it is the most violent reaction. If the reaction is so intense that it can spread within the mixture at a speed that is faster than the speed of sound then an explosion occurs.

If the proportions are allowed to differ more and more from this ideal the intensity of the reaction is reduced until the disproportion is so great that the reaction cannot start. This limit (and there are both an upper and a lower limit) is called the flammability limit.

An example would be ether:

	LOWER FLAMMABILITY LIMIT	STOICHIOMETRIC CONCENTRATION	UPPER FLAMMABILITY LIMIT
Ether & Air	2%	3.4%	34%
Ether & Oxygen	2%	14%	82%

Obviously, in oxygen (as opposed to air), there is a greater presence of oxidising agent and there is absence of nitrogen. The nitrogen acts by inhibiting the reaction, diluting the constituents and by absorbing some of the energy released. In general the risk of a reaction violent enough to case an explosion with vapours seen in anaesthetic practice is only present if the oxygen concentration is greater than that in room air.

---

10. WHAT METHODS ARE AVAILABLE ON THE STANDARD ANAESTHETIC MACHINE TO STOP THE DELIVERY OF A HYPOXIC GAS MIXTURE?

> ⊃ As with most questions that relate to the flow of gas through the machine or through a circuit the best way of dealing with this is to start at the wall and follow the gas flow through the machine to the patient.

1. Although the provision of the piped medical gases is not the responsibility of the anaesthetist it should be noted that there are specific regulations that control this supply, and its maintenance (HTM 22 in the UK).
2. The wall fitting for pipeline supply consists of a Schrader socket with an indexed collar. The socket is fixed to the flexible hose, and can only be removed by a service engineer. It is also designed so it cannot be attached to the wrong hose by accident. This is then permanently attached to the hose with a stainless steel ferrule.
3. The flexible non-compressible hose is colour coded along its whole length to prevent accidental misconnection if the hose is shortened. Although there are cases of cross-connection or errors in manufacturing (connecting the oxygen socket to the blue nitrous oxide hose) these have generally been minimised by tighter quality control and separation of the different assembly lines during manufacturing.
4. The machine end of the hose is permanently attached to a non-interchangeable connection consisting of a probe with gas-specific sized shoulders and a nut that can be connected to the machine with a spanner (known as a 'NIST', non-interchangeable screw threaded connection).
5. Methods to ensure the correct connection of the cylinder supply including the pin-index system are discussed elsewhere in the book.
6. The risk of leakage within the machine pipework is minimised by using gas-tight connections, either compression fittings, sealing washers or tapered threads.
7. Many machines feature secondary regulators that reduce the pressure within the machine to just below pipeline pressure (420 kPa) so that any fluctuation in the pipeline pressure is smoothed out.
8. The flowmeter bank on UK anaesthetic machines has to conform to BS 4272, so that the knobs must be labelled with the gas that they control, and the oxygen knob must be the largest and must project more than 2 mm proud of the other knobs. The oxygen knob is furthermore always placed on the left.
9. The flowmeters themselves have a number of features that help ensure accuracy, and so avoid the delivery of a hypoxic mixture. The bobbin has fins cut into its upper surface to make it spin, and so reduce the risk of sticking. There is also a conductive strip or coating on the inside of the tube to reduce the build-up of electrostatic charges and this also helps minimise sticking. The tubes are so designed that the bobbin cannot be hidden at the top of the tube.

10. All machines now must have an anti-hypoxia device linked to the flowmeters. The most commonly seen is a mechanical connection between the oxygen and nitrous oxide flowmeter knobs that ensures that it is impossible to dial a nitrous oxide: oxygen ratio of more than 3: 1 (i.e. an oxygen of 25%). This does not however consider any of the other gases attached or changes in the supply pressure.
11. Machines are fitted with an oxygen failure device.
12. Despite the left placement of the oxygen flowmeter, there is a risk of hypoxic delivery if there is a crack in one of the other flowmeters if the oxygen flows into the back bar on the left, before the inflow of the other gases. Therefore the gas from the oxygen flowmeter is ducted so that it enters the back bar downstream of the other gases.

---

11. HOW DOES AN OXYGEN DISCONNECT ALARM WORK?

⊃ **Oxygen failure alarms were initially introduced when the oxygen supply was provided by cylinders to reduce the risks of hypoxia due to emptying of these cylinders. Even with the almost universal use of nearly uninterrupted pipeline supply of oxygen it is still a requirement under British Standard for anaesthetic machines to be fitted with an oxygen failure alarm.**

The alarm is auditory (of at least 7 seconds duration and a specific minimum volume), and is powered by the oxygen supply itself to activate when the oxygen supply pressure falls to 200 kPa. It should also cut off the supply of the now hypoxic fresh gas flow from the patient and replace this with air either from an air supply or from the room.

A common oxygen failure device relies on a spring-loaded piston that is moved by the action of oxygen pressure on a diaphragm. As the supply pressure starts to fail (at 260 kPa) the piston is moved back by the spring, opening an auxiliary gas channel allowing gas to pass through the oxygen failure whistle sounding the alarm. This will continue to sound until the supply pressure fails to 40.5 kPa. As the pressure continues to fall (200 kPa) the piston moves further and finally is pulled onto a seating magnet that closes off the fresh gas flow by closing the cut-off valve. The fresh gas flow passes out through the pressure relief valve. This final movement also opens the air inspiratory valve and allow the patient (if not paralysed) to breath room air.

Working of a typical oxygen supply failure device

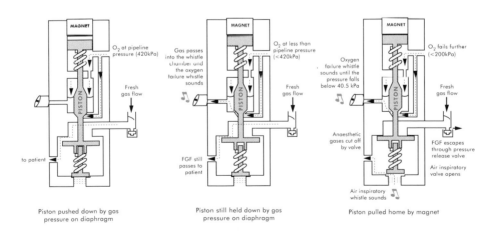

75

12. WHAT IS THE DIFFERENCE BETWEEN DECONTAMINATION, DISINFECTION AND STERILISATION?

⊃ **Anaesthetists commonly use reusable equipment and the methods adopted to ensure their safety is a fair topic for an examiner.**

Decontamination is the removal of infected material, and involves thorough cleaning and scrubbing. It makes the object more acceptable both bacteriologically and aesthetically. Detergents are generally used and after decontamination the object may be said to be 'clean'.

Disinfection involves the removal or killing of most of the infective organisms on the object. However there are resistant form of organisms such as spores that are NOT disabled by disinfection. It is adequate for many purposes, and avoids the use of high temperatures and pressures.

Sterilisation is the killing of all organisms including the resistant forms (spores) except prions (e.g. CJD), which are resistant to all forms of sterilisation. It may involve high temperatures and pressures, or chemical means.

It should be noted that these descriptions relate to the treatment of infectious matter, but has no indication about the removal or neutralisation of chemical contaminants.

---

13. HOW DO YOU PERFORM DECONTAMINATION, DISINFECTION AND STERILISATION?

⊃ Decontamination must be performed before either of the other two processes can be undertaken, as it removes the bulk of the infected material. This is important as the other procedures are only designed to be successful at treating small quantities of infected material.

Decontamination

Decontamination may be done in a medical version of the dishwasher, or by an ultrasonic washer. Most commonly it is done by hand scrubbing in detergent and hot water, followed by rinsing and air-drying.

Disinfection

Disinfection is most commonly performed by pasteurisation. This involves heating in a water bath (or in a low-pressure autoclave) and maintaining the required temperature for a set time. By not boiling plastic and rubber objects their usable life may be prolonged, as boiling tends to distort or perish them.

PASTEURISATION TIMES	
Temperature	Time
70°C	20 min
80°C	10 min
100°C	5 min

Boiling for a shorter period is equally successful if the object can withstand the heat.

It should be noted that the timing is from when the temperature of the water has returned to the required temperature after the last object has been inserted.

Chemical disinfection may be undertaken with 70% alcohol in water, chlorhexidine (either in 0.05% water with soaking for 30 minutes, or more rapidly by using 0.5% solution in 70% alcohol, in which case only 2 minutes is required), hypochlorite solutions ('bleach'), or gluteraldehyde (now replaced by less toxic alternatives).

Sterilisation

Sterilisation in theatres is most effectively and quickly performed by autoclaving. An autoclave is effectively a pressured steam cooker. The objects are placed in a gas tight

STERILISATION TIMES		
Pressure	Temperature	Time
15 psi	122°C	30 min
20 psi	126°C	10 min
30 psi	134°C	3 min

chamber and steam is pumped into and around the chamber raising the temperature and pressure. The time required depends on the temperature and the pressure. Chemical markers (such as the brown stripes on the tape of sterile supply bags) help ascertain that the autoclaving has been adequate.

Rubber and plastic items may be damaged by autoclaving, or may only last for a number of cycles before they must be disposed of, and many other items are not suitable for the rigors of the process.

Other techniques include low-pressure steam (at less than atmospheric pressure) used for delicate items, formaldehyde and ethylene oxide which can be used to sterilise whole anaesthetic machines.

Most disposable equipment is sterilised by gamma irradiation at the manufacturer.

---

14. WHAT ARE ACCEPTABLE LEVELS FOR THEATRE POLLUTION? WHAT ORGANISATION DETERMINES THESE?

> ⊃ **This topic is becoming more popular as a viva question. Worth the revision time, therefore.**

With regard to the recommended levels of pollutants in theatre (paricularly relevant to anesthetic gases and vapours) there is legal requirement under a code of practice drawn up by the Health and Safety Commission (HSC, 1996), to control exposure levels of many pollutants including anaesthetic agents. Some of the recommended maximum levels of exposure (averaged over any 8 hour time period) are listed below:

MAXIMUM ANAESTHETIC POLLUTANT LEVELS RECOMMENDED BY THE HSC	
Pollutant	Maximum level (ppm)
Nitrous oxide	100
Halothane	10
Enflurane	50
Isoflurane	50

---

15. WHAT SAFETY PRECAUTIONS ARE NECESSARY WHEN WORKING WITH LASERS?

⊃ Lasers are classified according to their degree of hazard from Class 1 (the least dangerous) to Class 4 (most dangerous). Domestic lasers (CD players, laser printers) are safe either because of the wavelengths used and their low power. However all surgical lasers are Class 4, being inherently hazardous as they are specifically designed to damage tissue.

Safety precautions when working with lasers include:

- Hazard sign outside theatre (illuminated)
- Appropriate training for all staff
- A designated suitably equipped area with all exposed surfaces matt finished
- All instruments with matt finish
- No inflammable material in the vicinity of the patient or in the operating field
- All theatre staff must wear protective eye glasses, and protection for the patient's eyes and skin against stray laser light
- The laser theatre must be well ventilated with a suitable smoke extraction system
- Precautions against indiscriminate use of inflammable or explosive anaesthetic gases
- Remember the flammability of gases in the airway when lasers are used. The old methods of wrapping ET tubes in foil or using saline soaked swabs have given way to the use of articulated metal tubes

CLINICAL ANAESTHESIA

NOTES ON THE CLINICAL VIVA

The clinical viva is unique in its organisation. Each of the examiners' information sheets contains three topics; a clinical scenario, a critical incident and a further clinical topic (which is not necessarily related to the previous questions). It is usual to be asked questions on all three areas but occasionally, time will not allow progress onto the third. In the examples that follow, each specimen viva is broken up into its component parts as an illustrative exercise. The examiners' notes on the critical incident are brief and there will therefore be a degree of variability in the way these events are introduced.

EXAMPLE 1

Scenario
A 54-year-old man presents for the repair of an inguinal hernia under GA as a day case. He is a smoker and admits to occasional chest pain on exercise for which his GP has prescribed a GTN spray. His ECG is normal apart from occasional unifocal ventricular ectopics and he is normotensive.

⊃ **Discussion will follow from the presentation of the scenario and will be directed by the examiner.**

You will be asked to consider the technique you would use, whether the ECG findings are important and the significance of ischaemic heart disease with respect to the conduct of anaesthesia. Usual day case criteria must be applied – ask about other features in the history (e.g. angina at rest? crescendo pattern? which would make the procedure undesirable). In the absence of any other factors, choose a cautious GA technique – propofol, opioid and volatile with a field block. Watch monitors for adverse events and avoid hypotension. In reality, there will be patients such as this served up every day across the country and basic principles of good anaesthetic practice apply (e.g. preoxygenation). This scenario often leads into a critical arrhythmia on table.

CRITICAL INCIDENT – ARRHYTHMIA

You notice occasional ventricular extra systoles which rapidly progress to 1 in 4 beats.

What do you do?

The sequence should be:

- Stop surgery
- 100% oxygen
- Check end tidal CO_2/respiratory pattern/oxygenation
- Keep watching ECG and measure BP
- Prepare cardiac drugs

This situation will now be examiner-directed and often leads on to the development of VT, then VF: you will be expected to know and follow the Broad Complex Tachycardia and VF algorithms as appropriate. Competence and safe practice are paramount in these situations and remember to keep the patient asleep when cardiac output is restored, after which a CCU bed should be sought. Finally, explain to the relatives and document the proceedings. In this example *viva*, the further clinical topic is directly related to the previous material.

FURTHER CLINICAL TOPIC

How would you assess the presence of ischaemic heart disease preoperatively?

⊃ **Clinically, and especially from the history, in the first instance. A chest X-ray is not useful unless failure is present.**

The electrocardiogram

This is useful, but only shows established changes and may be normal in the presence of ischaemic heart disease (IHD). However features of ischaemia include:

Features of old myocardial infarction

- ST depression
- Q waves } in affected leads
- T wave inversion

Features of existing ischaemia

- ST depression, commonly laterally
- Poor R wave progression through the anterior leads

Exercise electrocardiography

- Chest pain accompanied by > 2 mm ST depression is considered diagnostic of IHD
- Drop in blood pressure is suggestive of IHD

Thallium scanning

This uses injected thallium-201, which is taken up into cardiac muscle in proportion to the degree of perfusion. The isotope is detected with a gamma camera, demonstrating perfused areas, which can be scarred or ischaemic. The distinction is made by injecting a coronary vasodilator, such as dipyridamole; if an area is reversibly ischaemic, it will dilate and light up after administration of dipyridamole. It may then be appropriate to revascularise such areas before elective surgery.

Echocardiography

1. Abnormalities of wall motion indicate ischaemia or scarring. These are:

- Hypokinesis
- Akinesis
- Dyskinesis
- Reduced systolic thickening

2. Global dysfunction indicates a more severe disorder, and is represented by:

- End-diastolic dimension
- Ejection fraction, which can also be detected on multiple uptake gated acquisition (MUGA) which uses technetium-99 labelled red cells. This is not a first-line investigation for IHD

Holter 24-hour ST segment monitoring

This is an increasingly used investigation, observing as it does the pattern of ST morphology over an extended period. Holter monitoring was originally employed for the detection of arrhythmias. It has been found to be a highly significant predictor of postoperative cardiac events.

Pulmonary Artery Monitoring

While IHD causes decreased ventricular compliance, increased left ventricular end diastolic pressure and elevated wedge pressure, it is not an investigation routinely employed in this context.

As a continuation, the examiner may ask 'How common is ischaemic heart disease and what clinical features are suggestive of its presence?'

Lunn and Mushin described the prevalence of cardiovascular disease in the general surgical population as follows:

Age	**40–50:**	6%
Age	**50–60:**	23%
Age	**60–70:**	45%
Age	**over 70:**	100%

History of myocardial infarction is an obvious feature, as is angina pectoris. However, silent ischaemia is three times as common as angina; it occurs in the morning more than the afternoon, in the elderly, and in diabetics. Other risk factors include:

- Tobacco consumption
- Hypertension
- Obesity
- Family history
- High cholesterol – although this is becoming increasingly controversial

Other more subtle symptoms can be equally important. These include features of congestive cardiac failure:

- Coughing on lying flat
- Unexplained insomnia and nocturia
- Unexplained tachycardia or arrhythmias
- Dyspnoea accompanying angina, which is pathognemonic of transient left ventricular failure
- Chronic fatigue

EXAMPLE 2

Scenario
A woman of 36 presents for a laparoscopic cholecystectomy. She weighs 140 kg and has a BMI of 36. There are no other features of relevance in the history.

⊃ **The patient obviously fits the definition of morbid obesity and the questioning will revolve around the definition of Body Mass Index (weight in kg divided by height in metres – squared) and the attendant problems of anaesthesia in this group of patients.**

Obesity is increasing in the surgical population, and occurs in the female whose fat comprises more than 30% of her body weight, and in men when more than 25% of the body weight is fat.

Ideal body weight can be calculated by subtracting 100 (men) or 105 (women) from the height in cm.

For example: height 178: ideal weight = 178 – 100 = 78 kg

There are a number of ways of estimating obesity. The commonest is the Quetelet (BMI) index:

Body mass index (BMI)
<20   =   underweight
20 – 25   =   normal
25 – 30   =   overweight
30 – 35   =   obese
>35   =   morbidly obese

For example:
Height 1.782   =   3.17
Weight   =   77 kg
BMI   =   77 / 3.17   =   24 – in the normal range.

For example:
Height 1.502   =   2.25
Weight   =   95 kg
BMI   =   95 / 2.25   =   42 – morbid obesity.

Problems of anaesthesia should be organised by systems.

⊃ **The commonest problem in obesity is control of the airway, in this patient intubation is mandatory.**

Cardiovascular changes
▪ Increased cardiac output and cardiac work
▪ Hypertension (sleep hypoxaemia and increased erythropoeitin leading to polycythaemia; increased sympathetic activity; increased cardiac output; activated renin-angiotensin-aldosterone system)

- Increased stroke volume and left ventricular dimensions; this may proceed to LV failure
- Right ventricular hypertrophy and dilation, proceeding to RV failure
- Coronary artery disease (cholesterol, decreased high density lipoproteins, HDL) and ischaemic heart disease
- Cardiac arrhythmias (due to IHD, high catecholamines and increased cardiac work; fatty infiltration of cardiac muscle may also occur)

Respiratory changes

- Increased tendency to hypoxia: increased $\dot{V}O_2$ and CO_2 production, $\dot{V}/\dot{Q}$ mismatch and intrapulmonary shunt; patients also have high incidence of pulmonary disease
- Decreased pulmonary compliance, increasing the work of breathing (by 200% compared to the non-obese patient) and impairing breathing under anaesthesia
- Decreased functional residual capacity (FRC); also a shunt of 25% may be expected under GA
- Postoperative hypoxia is more common in obese patients
- Gastro-intestinal changes
- Gastro-oesophageal reflux (present in 75% of obese patients)
- Liver disease; fatty change and gallstones

Pharmacological changes

- Reduced fraction of total body water
- Increased adipose compartment
- Increased cardiac output
- Increased free fatty acids, triglycerides, cholesterol and α-1 acid glycoprotein

Other changes

- Difficult venous access
- Positioning: in extreme cases, may need two operating tables

CRITICAL INCIDENT – HYPOXIA

Your patient suddenly becomes hypoxic in the middle of the operation, saturation falls from 95% to 88%.

> ⊃ A modified ABC approach is useful here. Is the airway clear? Has the ETT become displaced? Is the patient being ventilated effectively? Is there good cardiac output? Check systematically back from ETT to anaesthetic machine and change to 100% oxygen plus hand ventilation in the first instance, restoring the volatile as soon as the situation allows.

Make the surgeon deflate the abdomen. Consider:

- Endobrochial intubation
- Bronchospasm

- Aspiration
- Mechanical blockage/inadequate tidal respiration
- Muscle relaxation
- Other causes, such as emboli

Your performance in this question will largely depend on the organisation and safe conduct of the incident. Remember record keeping at the resolution of the crisis. Usually, this situation will be directed to a misplacement of the ETT into a main bronchus, which is readily remedied.

FURTHER CLINICAL TOPIC

How do you calculate the amount of fluid needed for resuscitation in a burnt patient?

> ⊃ **There are several methods but familiarity is expected with only one.**

The Muir and Barclay formula deals with the so-called 'shock' phase of the injury, the first 36 hours, and dictates replacement therapy, dealing with colloid (Albumin solution), and crystalloid, as well as blood. This depends on calculation of body surface burn (BSB) in percent, and body weight (BW) in kg. It must be calculated from the time of injury, not from time of admission.

1. Colloid: (BW × %BSB) / 2 = ml per block.

                      Blocks at 4, 4, 4, 6, 6, 12 hours post injury.

2. Crystalloid: (1.5 × BW) ml/hr.

3. Blood: 50 ml/%BSB.

To monitor progress, many would say that a pulmonary artery catheter is essential, and that the problems of infection from lines are outweighed by the advantages of reliable data on the patient's cardiovascular status. A urinary catheter is essential. The static plasma deficit allows hour-to-hour progress to be calculated based on haematocrit, and is a useful tool. It requires a knowledge of the patient's calculated normal blood volume (BV).

To calculate blood volume:

- Adult: 7% body weight, or 70 ml/kg
- Child: 80 ml/kg
- Neonate: 90 ml/kg
- Deficit = $BV - \dfrac{(BV \times normal\ Hct)}{Observed\ Hct}$

EXAMPLE 3

Scenario
You are called to Accident and Emergency to see a 76-year-old man with burns. What would make you suspect the presence of an inhalational injury?

⊃ Consider the direct effects of burns on the airway as well as the metabolic consequences such as carboxyhaemoglobinaemia. Inhalational injury must be considered if there is a history of entrapment in an enclosed space, and is less likely, though not impossible, with an electrical burn.

Other indicators of inhalational injury are:

- Facial involvement of burns
- Burnt nares, soot in nose
- Stridor, which is an indication for immediate tracheal intubation
- Evidence at laryngoscopy

Retrospective carbon monoxide (CO) estimation

The lab co-oximeter will quantify CO levels (but, of considerable importance, the bedside oximeter will not, and cannot distinguish carboxyhaemoglobin (COHb) from oxyhaemoglobin. A patient whose haemoglobin is apparently 99% saturated according to a pulse oximeter may be dying of hypoxia). If the time of injury is known, the exposure levels of CO may be calculated from a nomogram and inhalation injury inferred if a high level is calculated. Presence of COHb is also associated with inhalation of other toxins such as cyanide produced by burning plastics.

The treatment of carboxyhaemoglobinaemia depends on displacement of the CO from the Hb molecule to which it is very tightly bound. The half-life of COHb is 250 minutes in air, 50 minutes in 100% O_2, and 22 minutes in a hyperbaric chamber at 2.5 atmospheres. Getting the patient into a chamber fast enough is another matter.

⊃ A low threshold for intubation and ventilation is recommended. HDU or ITU care should be considered if there is reasonable suspicion of serious smoke inhalation as the situation may deteriorate rapidly.

CRITICAL INCIDENT – FAILED INTUBATION

You are unable to visualise the larynx when performing a rapid sequence intubation. What will you do?

⊃ This is a common question. You must have a prepared plan – 'Failed intubation drill'.

Failed intubation occurs with an incidence of 1: 3,000 in the general population, but rises to 1: 300 in the third trimester of pregnancy. The first such drill was first described by Tunstall in connection with failed obstetric intubation, and has been modified many times since. It is also appropriate for other situations where the airway is at risk of soiling with gastric contents. Oxygenation is paramount.

The key points are:

- Get help quickly
- Recognition: if misplacement has occurred, this is seen with a capnogram
- Oxygenation is more important than repeated attempts to intubate

MANAGEMENT OF FAILED INTUBATION

Call for help. If cricoid pressure has been applied it should not be released. Tilt the table head down. Suction pharynx as required. Insert oral airway and institute bag and mask ventilation with 100% oxygen. If this is difficult a two person effort may be required, one to maintain the airway, the other to squeeze the reservoir bag. If ventilation is satisfactory consider waking the patient up. In an emergency (Caesarean section for foetal distress, for example) maintain cricoid pressure and allow spontaneous respiration to return. Continue anaesthesia via a face mask.

If ventilation is difficult try inserting a laryngeal mask airway. If ventilation is impossible both with a conventional mask and through a laryngeal mask airway, consider severe laryngeal spasm as a cause. If this has been excluded perform an emergency cricothyroid puncture with a 16 or 14 G cannula. Once in the trachea remove the needle and connect the catheter to a 2 ml syringe. Discard the plunger and insert a size 7.0 mm endotracheal tube (Portex) connector inside the syringe, attach this to a catheter mount and anaesthetic circuit.

FURTHER CLINICAL TOPIC
What methods are available for pain relief in labour?

⊃ **An overview is required here.**

Transcutaneous Electrical Nerve Stimulation (TENS)
This works by means of the gate theory and is often perfectly adequate for mothers in early and sometimes advanced labour. Electrodes are placed on dermatomes corresponding to the source of pain, in other words to the uterus, T10 – L1. Low frequency high amplitude stimulation of the Ab fibres closes the gate.

Inhalational Methods
These operate at a cortical and thalamic level, and affect conscious level. The effect is however very transient and inhalational agents will reach the foetus. In the past, this has included methoxyflurane and trichloroethylene, both now unavailable. This leaves Entonox, which is 50% nitrous oxide in oxygen. The cylinders are blue with blue and white shoulders and are available in sizes D (500 litres) F (2000 litres) and G (5000 litres). Delivery is from a demand valve operated by maternal inspiration. Only about 50% of mothers who use Entonox derive adequate analgesia, and there are two other particular problems. Firstly the use of the demand valve requires some teaching, and the parturient must be co-ordinating her inhalation with the

beginning of the contraction since the analgesic effect takes 45 seconds to be maximal. Secondly, there is a tendency to hyperventilation, which reduces oxygen delivery to the foetus. Isoflurane may be used for this in the future as it has modest analgesic properties.

Intramuscular Opioids
Pethidine 150 mg, with further doses of 100 mg up to three times, may be administered by Midwifery staff without a doctor's prescription. The main objection to the use of pethidine is that, once administered, it accumulates in the foetus and causes neonatal respiratory depression. Metabolites of pethidine are detectable for a prolonged period post delivery. Of all the available opiates, pethidine is probably the least effective as an analgesic. It is short acting and has atropine-like effects.

Patient-controlled intravenous analgesia (PCA) is used to good effect in some centres as an alternative to intramuscular analgesia.

Regional Analgesia
Modern thinking is that this is the safest and most effective means of providing analgesia, from the point of view of the mother and the foetus. Indeed it has considerable advantages over other forms in certain situations, e.g. pre-eclampsia, where it assists in the control of blood pressure. Also in multiple births, where the second twin is delivered in better condition, and where intervention is anticipated, when a long labour may be made more comfortable and the hazards of general anaesthesia avoided.

There are only two situations when a regional technique absolutely must not be used. These are maternal refusal and bleeding disorder. Sepsis, hypovolaemia (and the risk of hypovolaemia), and urgency of delivery are all relative contraindications. Neither aspirin nor previous back surgery are contraindications.

EXAMPLE 4

Scenario
On your pre-operative ward round you visit an elderly lady who has come in for a knee replacement. She has suffered from rheumatoid arthritis for several years. What factors do you consider when making your assessment of her fitness for anaesthesia?

⊃ **Rheumatoid arthritis (RA) affects 3% of the population, in a ratio of 3:1 Female:Male. It is therefore a common condition and many affected patients present for surgery and anaesthesia.**

Rheumatoid arthritis has an insidious onset from the 4th decade of life onwards. Seropositive (IgM) RA is more common in people with HLA-DR4 than in the general population, and hence there is a genetic influence.

⊃ **It is best to divide your answer into consideration of each physiological system in turn.**

Cardiovascular considerations
10% have a pericarditis, which is often asymptomatic. 30% have a small pericardial effusion; rheumatoid nodules may form in the cardiac conducting tissues. The vasculitis may cause Raynaud's phenomenon and nail bed, cranial, coronary and mesenteric infarcts. There is a chronic anaemia (a haemoglobin of 10 g/dl is common), which correlates inversely with the erythrocyte sedimentation rate (ESR). This is worsened by the inevitable non-steroidal anti-inflammatory drug (NSAID) therapy these patients are prescribed.

Respiratory considerations
Pleural rubs, nodules and effusions are common, but rarely serious. Parenchymal disease is common if you look for it, but fibrosing alveolitis develops in only 2%, although it has a poor prognosis. RA with pneumoconiosis is Caplan's syndrome, a disease of massive confluent pulmonary rheumatoid nodules. Chest wall compliance decreases due to stiff costovertebral and intervertebral joints.

Musculoskeletal considerations
There will be a symmetrical arthropathy involving interphalangeal joints, metacarpophalangeal joints, wrists, knees and ankles. Temporomandibular joints may be affected, reducing mouth opening, and RA affecting the cricoarytenoid joints, although described, is extremely rare. The terminal interphalangeal joint is never affected. Morning stiffness is characteristic, as is a return of symptoms in the evening – "vesperal" stiffness. Of most concern is involvement of the occipito-atlanto-axial joint (OAA), and especially of subluxation (atlas slides forward on axis) in flexion, where ligamentous laxity and erosion of the odontoid peg exist. Identification of this is notoriously difficult. 25% will have radiological evidence, while only 5% will have problems. Cervical myelopathy is a serious consideration. Neck involvement is late, and affects the top end – the OAA complex – in contrast to osteoarthritis, which affects the bottom end.

Renal considerations

Amyloid deposition may occur and this may lead to renal impairment made obvious on electrolyte results.

Other considerations

Peptic ulceration is common. Sjögren's syndrome (keratoconjuntivitis sicca), scleritis and uveitis may be present. The patient will have been on steroids and other immunosuppresants. Gold causes marrow suppression, pulmonary fibrosis and both renal and hepatic impairment. Infections, both intra- and extra-articular, are common.

This viva topic may be directed in a particular direction by the examiner. For example, as a further question: Her haemoglobin result is 8.9 g/dl. What do you think of that?

⊃ **Haemoglobin value may be explained by anaemia of chronic disease.**

The common picture is normocytic, normochromic anaemia, low serum iron concentration, low serum transferring concentration and saturation, high serum ferritin concentration.

⊃ **What is the physiological response to chronic anaemia?**

- Increased 2,3-DPG levels that facilitate oxygen delivery to tissues
- Increase erythropoietin production
- Decreased blood viscosity, concomitant recruitment, increased oxygen extraction, increased cardiac output

⊃ **What haematinics do you know?**

- Iron supplements (IV better than oral)
- Recombinant Human erythropoietin

CRITICAL INCIDENT – WRONG BLOOD

What happens if the wrong blood transfusion is given to a patient?

⊃ **This will largely depend on the extent of the antigenic mis–match and how quickly the mistake is recognised.**

Mild signs:

- Fever
- Rash – (seen in 2% of all transfusion recipients)

More severe signs:

- Cardiovascular: Chest pain, hypotension
- Respiratory: Dyspnoea, pulmonary oedema,
- Renal: Oliguria, haemoglobinuria
- Coagulopathy, haemoglobinuria, haemoglobinaemia

Many of these features may not be apparent in an anaesthetised patient. Incidence of acute intravascular haemolysis from ABO incompatibility is 1 death in 34,000 transfused.

Management of transfusion reactions

> ⊃ **Divide your answer into therapy and investigation.**

Therapy for suspected haemolytic transfusion reaction
- Stop transfusion. Keep IV open with normal saline
- Give 100% oxygen
- All principles of basic life support apply – Airway, Breathing, Circulation
- Catheterise to monitor urine output
- Diuretic therapy –frusemide or consider mannitol
- Monitor CVP
- Treat electrolyte imbalances such as hyperkalaemia
- Treat acid-base imbalances with bicarbonate
- Blood component therapy to support disseminated intravascular coagulation.
- Use rematched blood if red cells are essential. No increased risk of second haemolytic reactions

Investigation
- Double check the label of blood unit and patient's ID with other identifiers
- Take 40 ml blood for:
  - Blood bank to report the plasma haemoglobin and direct antiglobulin test
  - U&E, Coagulation profile, Full blood count and film
  - Bacteriology for blood cultures
- Repeat compatibility test with pre- and post-transfusion samples
- Blood packs and giving sets examined for bacterial contamination
- ECG
- Urine for microscopy

FURTHER CLINICAL TOPIC

How can you assess the severity of a patient's pain?

Important aspects of pain
- Functional impairment
- Quality of life (as perceived by patient and not the assessor)
- Pain behaviour

Pain has three components
- Sensory discriminative
- Motivational affective
- Cognitive evaluative

Single dimensional scores
Visual Analogue Scores
- Able to use in children > 7 years
- Good for current pain, not good for "remembered" pain

- Extremes are made absolute
- Does not regard other components of pain

Verbal Numerical Scale
- Whaley and Wong Facial Scoring for children

Multi dimensional scores
- Wisconsin Brief Pain Questionnaire
  - 17 questions, self-administered
  - Location, pain drawing, incorporates verbal numerical scale
  - Interference of activities of daily living

- McGill Pain Questionnaire

3 main parts to this popular questionnaire:
  - Descriptive scale for **p**resent **p**ain **i**ntensity (PPI)
    - Numbers assigned to 5 adjectives mild (1) to excruciating (5)
  - Drawing of human figure to mark areas of pain
  - Pain rating index
    - Patient selects adjectives from 20 categories reflecting sensory, affective and cognitive components

Functional assessment
Disability
- Sickness Impact profile
- Health Assessment Questionnaire
- Pain Disability Index

Psychological indicators and quality of life
- Beck Depression Inventory

EXAMPLE 5

Scenario

A 48-year-old male patient presents for varicose vein surgery. He has a history of smoking 20-30 cigarettes a day since age 14. On examination you find scattered wheeze and odd coarse crepitations in all lung fields. He declares himself well but has a 'fruity' smoker's cough. Should patients such as this be encouraged to give up smoking before anaesthesia when surgery is not essential?

⊃ **Basically-yes! There are immediate, short-term and long-term reasons to cease smoking prior to anaesthesia.**

Smokers are more likely to desaturate in recovery, as are the passive-smoking children of smoking parents.

Immediate reasons: These relate to oxygen delivery

The half-life of carboxyhaemoglobin (COHb) is 250 minutes in room air; COHb displaces oxygen from haemoglobin, but is not detected by pulse oximetry, which reads COHb as HbO. A heavy smoker (60/day) may have a COHb of 15%, so that his or her HbO is, at best, 85%. A bedside pulse oximetry reading of 92% clearly indicates much worse hypoxia in such a case. This has obvious implications for oxygen delivery. Nicotine is a sympathetic stimulant, so there is a chance of accelerated cardiac function in the context of reduced oxygen delivery. Abstinence from smoking for 12 hours restores oxygen carriage to that of the non-smoker.

Short term reasons: These mostly relate to pulmonary function

Smokers have increased pulmonary secretions and airway sensitivity. They also have small airway narrowing and a tendency to $\dot{V}/\dot{Q}$ mismatch. They have up to a 6-fold increase in atelectasis and pneumonia compared to non-smokers, and an increased incidence of laryngo- and bronchospasm. These effects are abolished after a period of abstinence from smoking of 6–8 weeks. In addition, nicotine induces hepatic enzymes and smokers have an increased clearance of certain sedative and anaesthetic drugs.

Long term reasons: These relate to malignancy and cardiovascular function

Smokers have a tendency to thrombo-embolic disease and have increased coronary vascular resistance. Tobacco smoke contains at least 43 carcinogens. The risk of pulmonary malignancy in a reformed smoker after 7 years of abstinence falls to that of the non-smoking population.

CRITICAL INCIDENT – HYPERTENSION

You are called to recovery to see a patient who has had a laparoscopic cholecystectomy (not your patient) because his blood pressure is 190/100.

> ↻ There are several possible causes for this. The commonest cause in previously healthy patients is severe pain but other causes especially CO_2 retention should be sought before this is confirmed as the cause. As always with any recovery scenario use an ABC approach first to exclude airway, respiratory or cardiovascular problems that require immediate attention.

The major causes of hypertension are all mediated via an increase in sympathetic tone.

- Pre-existing hypertension – especially if routine medication has been omitted
- Pain
- Anxiety (precipitated sometimes by inadequate reversal of muscle relaxation)
- Carbon dioxide retention
- Hypothermic vasoconstriction
- Hypoxia
- Pyrexia
- Drugs
  - ketamine
  - myocardial stimulants
  - vasoconstrictors
- Endocrine disease
  - thyrotoxicosis
  - pheochromocytoma
  - carcinoid syndrome
- Raised ICP
- Spinal cord trauma

In the absence of respiratory insufficiency it is likely that extra analgesia will result in the values settling but keep the other reasons in mind and explain your differential diagnosis to the examiner.

FURTHER CLINICAL TOPIC

What are the complications associated with epidural analgesia in labour? How are these complications managed?

> ↻ Complications may be broadly divided into early and late. As a generalisation, the early complications are common and easily managed; it is the late complications, which are rarer and more serious.

Early complications

1. *Failure*: This may occur up to 4%. Re-siting will be necessary.
2. *Unilaterality (a one-sided block)*: This may be due to the catheter emerging from the paravertebral foramen rather than lying in the epidural space. This may happen up in to 15%, but is less common where opioids are used in the epidural mixture. An over-long catheter may extrude through an intervertebral foramen and any local anaesthetic introduced will tend to spill out of the epidural space. If adjustment of the length of catheter in the space does not resolve this, the catheter should be resited.
3. *Dural tap*: A rate of 0.5% is taken as acceptable. Young people with a dural tear are likely to develop post dural puncture headache (PDPH). The epidural blood patch is the definitive treatment for PDPH; rest and epidural infusion probably just delay onset. Some PDPH will resolve spontaneously. For this reason a blood patch should not be offered until 24 hours after the onset of the headache. The long-term risk of PDPH concerns dural traction due to the reduced volume of CSF, with the traction causing a subdural haematoma. A blood patch should therefore not be delayed beyond the 24 hour point. Avoidance of pushing in the second stage of labour makes no difference to the incidence or the severity of the PDPH.
4. *Total spinal anaesthetic*: This is where the intended epidural dose goes into the subaracnoid space. For this to happen, a large dose of local anaesthetic must be delivered, such as 15 ml of 0.5% bupivacaine; there will be progressive ascending weakness, hypotension, respiratory failure, and, with the airway protective reflexes obtunded, a risk of aspiration. Management involves early recognition and resuscitation; intubation and ventilation, elevation of the feet with uterine displacement, vasopressors, and fluids will be required. However, in epidural analgesia for labour, very low concentrations of local anaesthetic are used. It has been shown that if the total epidural top-up of 15 ml of 0.1% bupivacaine, which is intended to be given by the midwife, is instead placed in the subarachnoid space, a dense block to T4 ensues; for a total spinal to happen, the amount of bupivacaine needs to be very much greater. It is possible to cause a total spinal with the amount of bupivacaine used for epidural Caesarean section.
5. *Inadvertent intravenous injection*: This causes cardiovascular toxicity. The cardiac collapse to central nervous system toxicity (CC/CNS) ratio dictates the relative safety of different agents; it compares the dose required to produce systemic CNS effects (oral tingling, depression of conscious level) to those levels required to produce cardiovascular effects. The CC/CNS ratio is 7: 1 for lidocaine but only 3: 1 for bupivacaine. Levo-Bupivacaine is beneficial because this ratio is increased. The treatment of local anaesthetic-induced arrhythmia is Bretylium, 7 mg/kg.
6. *Anaphylaxis*: This is very rare, since preservatives, which are the usual implicated component, are not used in spinal or epidural anaesthesia.
7. *Minor side effects*: These include a degree of sympathetic block, which should be treated with vasopressors; shivering, which is lessened by the addition of an opioid to the epidural mixture, and pruritis, caused by the opioid, which

8. *Complications due to misplacement of the epidural catheter or of the Tuohy needle*: There are a number of ways of misplacing the needle or the catheter, which may result in a subarachnoid block, a total spinal, a mixed block, or a subdural block. The latter is a delayed, but dense, block of sudden onset, which may spare the motor component. As can be seen, neither the aspiration test nor the test dose is either sensitive or specific.

Late complications

1. *Neurological – cord compression or ischaemia*. Spinal haematoma is very rare and can occur in the absence of a regional block. Inappropriate motor block, dense or prolonged, is an ominous sign. It is a neurosurgical emergency. Cord ischaemia is a complication of epidural anaesthesia in the elderly, not in the young.
2. *Neurological – single nerve palsies*. These are often indistinguishable from those caused by obstetric trauma. Cauda equina syndrome is a complication of spinal, not epidural, anaesthesia.
3. *Sepsis*.
4. *Bladder dysfunction*: Retention of urine and bladder dystonia. This is legally indefensible.
5. *Backache*: This is a frequent occurence, but is due in large part to the obstetrics, to posture (lithotomy) and to motor blockade. Local discomfort from the puncture site needs to be explained beforehand to the mother and is self-limiting.

EXAMPLE 6

Scenario
You have a patient on your list for thyroidectomy. A large goitre is obvious on examination. What considerations do you make?

⊃ **You should consider the possibility of an endocrine disturbance, the risk of a deformity of the airway (per- or post operatively), and the risk of existing or operatively-induced recurrent laryngeal nerve damage.**

The presence of goitre is consistent with hypo-, hyper-, or euthyroid function. Biochemical thyroid function testing is therefore mandatory. Briefly, the risks of hyperthyroidism are:

- Cardiac arrhythmias, especially tachycardia, and atrial and ventricular fibrillation
- Uncontrolled hypertension
- Cardiac ischaemia
- Excessive haemorrhage
- Thyroid 'storm'

The airway must be assessed clinically and with a thoracic inlet X-ray. This will reveal deviation or compression of the trachea, and allow planning of the means of airway control and anticipation of a difficult intubation; a smaller tube than usual will be needed, and elective tracheostomy has been described for massive goitre. The thoracic inlet is 10 × 5 cm and kidney-shaped, inclined 60° forwards and bounded by the first thoracic vertebra, the first ribs, and the manubrium. The integrity of the trachea may be dependent on support from the goitre, in which case tracheomalacia, with collapse of the trachea on inspiration, may occur postoperatively.

Ideally, the patient should be euthyroid and if difficult intubation is likely arrange all equipment close to hand, seek help in advance and consider fibreoptic (nasal or oral) airway instrumentation.

CRITICAL INCIDENT – FAILURE TO BREATHE

You are summoned by the recovery sister to see your postoperative laparotomy who is 'Not breathing too well, Doctor'.

⊃ **Immediate assessment of the severity of the problem is mandatory. Is there hypoxia? Is there cardiac output? Is the patient rousable? What is the respiratory pattern? Secure the airway, if necessary re-intubating – which will depend on circumstances. Only when the immediate situation is secure, should you think more about the causes.**

Causes of failure to breath adequately in the recovery room
Drugs
- Opioids
- Neuromuscular blockade – reversal

Respiratory
- Obstructed airway, blood, airway swelling

Physical
- Cold temperature

Neurological
- Cerebrovascular accident

Patient factors
- Elderly slow to metabolise drugs
- Hypotensiion (?post operative bleeding)

Urea and Electrolytes
- Hypokalaemia
- Obstructive Sleep Apnoea

Metabolic
- Myxoedema

FURTHER CLINICAL TOPIC

What criteria make a patient appropriate for day surgery?

> ⊃ **Day surgery may account for more than 50% of elective general surgery. Divide your answer firstly into discussion of appropriate surgical procedures; thereafter, discuss medical, surgical, and social exclusions.**

There are many procedures carried out as day cases, and the number is increasing – body wall procedures including hernia repair, varicose veins, circumcision, and removal of skin lesions; urological procedures such as cystoscopy, vasectomy and excision of epididymal cyst. Circumcision is best carried out with a penile block for analgesia that avoids the motor block seen with a caudal, which might prevent the patient returning home. Gynaecological procedures include hysteroscopy and dilatation and curettage, laparoscopy (including sterilisation) and termination of pregnancy. Ear, nose and throat work, which involves a large number of children, include myringotomy and grommet insertion and polypectomy. Most dentistry has almost always been done as day cases and is therefore not included here.

Medical exclusions
- Cardiac: severe ischaemic heart disease, advanced hypertension, congestive cardiac failure
- Bleeding disorders
- Diabetes mellitus
- Obesity with body mass index over 35 (this varies from hospital to hospital)
- Muscular disease
- Poorly controlled epilepsy

Surgical and anaesthetic exclusions

- Malignant hyperpyrexia susceptibility
- Previous anaphylactic reaction to anaesthesia
- Scoline apnoea is controversial

Social exclusions

- No transport, telephone or supervision for 24 hours

EXAMPLE 7

Scenario
A 60-year-old male patient with myotonia dystrophica appears on your list for cataract surgery. How would you conduct anaesthesia in a patient with the condition?

⊃ **Myotonia dystrophica is an autosomal dominant condition affecting men and women equally, and is also known as myotonic dystrophy, dystrophia myotonica, myotonia atrophica, and Steinert's Disease.**

Features
- Patient: this is a rare condition, inherited as an autosomal dominant with anticipation. There is wasting, frontal balding, diabetes, cataracts and mental retardation.
- Cardiovascular system: cardiac muscle is affected. Cardiac failure is the usual mode of death, in the sixth decade of life. Conduction defects are common.
- Respiratory system: pulmonary function is abnormal, and the CO_2 response curve is right-shifted.
- Musculoskeletal system: myotonia results in delayed release of contraction, as in a handshake, and is precipitated by cold, exercise, shivering, hyperkalaemia, suxamethonium (intubation may be impossible) and neostigmine.
- There are no associations with the renal system.

Conduct of anaesthesia
- The surgery is often for cataract removal. This begs to be done under local anaesthesia. Other surgical procedures may be required, as for the general population.
- Preoperatively: 24 hour ECG may indicate rhythm instability. Lung function and ECG are mandatory. Avoid all sedative premedication.
- Anaesthesia: Regional techniques are relatively contraindicated because of the profound weakness produced (acceptable for eye surgery, however). Thiopentone causes profound depression, but propofol less so. Because of the likelihood of bulbar involvement, as well as respiratory muscle weakness, intubation and ventilation are essential. Suxamethonium is a disaster; atracurium, allowed to wear off at the end to avoid using neostigmine, is the preferred form of muscle relaxation.
- Maintenance: volatile anaesthetic agents cause exaggerated negative inotropic effects. Opioids also have an enhanced effect.
- Postoperatively: Intensive Care is often required, because of cardiac instability and respiratory embarrassment. The risk of pulmonary aspiration is considerable.

CRITICAL INCIDENT – AIR EMBOLISM

When might you see a venous air embolus?

> ⊃ **This is one of the most significant complications of neurosurgery but can occur in any 'head up' head and neck operation. It occurs because the veins, which are at negative pressure, become open to air, which is subsequently entrained.**

The morbidity is related to the size of the embolus, which may be reduced by rapid detection. In most cases the embolus ends in the right ventricle, where it may compromise cardiac output if large enough. In cases of patent foramen ovale, a paradoxical embolus may occur with return of the embolus to vital tissue, which will include the brain because of gravity.

Nitrous oxide causes any air embolus to enlarge. The use of a stethoscope and a capnograph will allow early detection, with a 'mill wheel' murmur and a decrease in end-tidal CO_2. The latter is most reliably detected with the trend display on the capnograph, as the onset of a venous air embolus may be insidious.

You will inevitably be asked about management. The management of venous air embolus is directed at stopping any further embolism by flooding the operation site with saline and packs, and supporting the circulation with 100% oxygen and fluids, level the table if possible. Compression of the neck veins to raise venous pressure above atmospheric has been used. In some cases air may be retrieved from the right side of the heart if a central line is in place.

FURTHER CLINICAL TOPIC

How can the risk of recall during general anaesthesia be reduced?

> ⊃ **This may be divided into how you monitor the apparatus, and how you apply your pharmacological and physiological knowledge.**

Apparatus
- Check all apparatus before each operating list
- Check ventilator, breathing system and vaporiser before each case
- Ensure adequate servicing of equipment
- Equipment must then be rechecked frequently throughout anaesthesia to ensure adequacy of vaporiser filling, cylinder levels, tightness of connections
- If an intravenous technique is used then the function of the pump, the continuity of the infusion tubing and the continued positioning and functioning of the indwelling cannula must be checked

Resuscitation
All patients should be adequately resuscitated so that adequate anaesthesia is not inhibited by the need to avoid excessive cardiovascular depression.

Dose of Induction Agent
Use an adequate dose, which may be more than the sleep dose especially in young, unpremedicated patients.

Duration of Action of Induction Agent

Ensure adequate anaesthesia is present by other means before the effect of the induction agent wears off, particularly if intubation is achieved using non-depolarising muscle relaxants that have a relatively slower speed of onset than suxamethonium.

Difficult Intubation

Between intubation attempts the patient must not only be reoxygenated but anaesthesia must be continued by inhalational or intravenous means.

Nitrous Oxide-Oxygen

This combination alone is not an anaesthetic and supplemental agents must be used.

Opioids

Conventional doses of opioid do not ensure unconsciousness, and they should be used as part of a balanced technique.

Dose of Inhalational Agents

Use of expired agent concentration monitors can help ensure that the alveolar concentration of inhalational anaesthetic agents is adequate to ensure anaesthesia.

Reversal of Muscle Relaxants

Anaesthesia either by nitrous oxide or other means must be continued until there is objective evidence of the adequacy of reversal of muscle relaxants.

Amnesic Drugs

The use of benzodiazepines either pre- or intra-operatively has been suggested as an effective way to reduce conscious recall. Their use in this manner, however, remains somewhat controversial and is not recommended. Anterograde amnesia is unlikely to be produced by any benzodiazepine.

EXAMPLE 8

Scenario
You are asked to anaesthetise a patient with porphyria. What is the condition, and how will you conduct the anaesthetic?

⊃ There are two groups of porphyria; erythropoetic and hepatic. Anaesthesia does not induce erythropoetic forms. Discuss the condition first and then outline a technique that you would be prepared to administer.

The clinical effects of porphyria are due to overproduction of haem precursors, which are highly toxic, due to the overactivity of a small, readily induced enzyme. The enzyme is *d*-aminolaevulinic acid (ALA) synthetase, and the disease is due to a relative deficiency of another enzyme later on in the synthetic process, thus allowing accumulation of intermediate metabolites. The position of the deficient enzyme predicts the type of precursor to accumulate and the pattern of the disease. Smaller intermediates cross the blood-brain barrier and cause neuropsychiatric disturbance, while larger ones cause cutaneous manifestations.

The two important conditions are Acute Intermittent Porphyria (AIP) and Variegate Porphyria (VP). Both are inherited in an autosomal dominant form. Both are precipitated by induction of ALA synthetase by pregnancy, dieting, and drugs of importance such as barbiturates, steroids, sulphonamides and griseofulvin. Management of an attack involves analgesia, carbohydrate loading, beta-blockade, fluids and haematin solutions to suppress ALA synthetase activity.

- Acute Intermittent Porphyria: this is due to a deficiency of uroporphyrinogen I synthase, allowing accumulation of small metabolites: thus the picture is of abdominal pain, neuropathy, and psychosis. AIP is common in Scandinavia and diagnosis is made by finding ALA in the urine.
- Variegate Porphyria: this is due to deficiency of Protoporphyrinogen oxidase, allowing accumulation of large metabolites; cutaneous manifestations of rash and necrosis occur in addition to neurological phenomena, and diagnosis is made by finding porphyrins in the stool.

Conduct of anaesthesia
Anaesthesia: regional techniques are safe. Barbiturates are absolutely contraindicated. A safe anaesthetic includes: propofol, fentanyl, isoflurane in N_2O, atracurium, droperidol, neostigmine and atropine.

Postoperatively: adequate analgesia is essential to avoid precipitating an acute attack.

CRITICAL INCIDENT – PNEUMOTHORAX

⊃ **This topic may be introduced in a variety of ways – as a change in airway pressure during IPPV, or as a sudden event in a trauma call to A and E, to give a couple of examples.**

⊃ **Commonly, the discussion will revolve around the physical signs – reduced air entry and tracheal shift and you will be expected to differentiate between the urgent (tension) situation with cardiovascular compromise and the less urgent situation when a little more time may be taken. After diagnosis (which might need a small needle diagnostic puncture to release tension) placement of a chest drain is required, unless a very trivial pneumothorax is present.**

The site should be chosen as follows:

Emergency: Second interspace, mid-clavicular line
Less urgent: Fifth interspace, mid-axillary line

An underwater seal is necessary, although temporarily a one-way Heimlich type valve will suffice.

FURTHER CLINICAL TOPIC

What are the hazards of laparoscopy?

⊃ **The laparoscopic approach used to be used almost exclusively by gynaecologists, but is now widely used by general, thoracic and even cardiac surgeons.**

These can be considered under complications of any general anaesthetic, and those specific to laparoscopy. Specific to laparoscopy are:

- Pulmonary oedema from fluid and the head-down position, which causes autotransfusion.
- The commonest structure impaled by the laparoscope is the distended stomach (1:200) so consider passing a nasogastric tube and aspirating the stomach if induction has involved prolonged manual ventilation by bag and mask. Regurgitation of gastric contents is also a risk.
- Insufflation is the most hazardous part of the procedure; 1:2000 patients have a demonstrable gas embolism, so beware high insufflating pressure and low flow. Signs of gas embolism are arrhythmia, hypotension, cyanosis and cardiac arrest. The safest technique involves the use of CO_2 for the pneumoperitoneum rather than N_2O, because CO_2 is more soluble and if an embolism occurs, it will resolve faster. You should watch the indicators on the insufflating machine continuously during inflation, and beware

pressure over 3 kPa or total volume insufflated exceeding 5 litres. Avoid excessive head down tilt, and always be prepared for laparotomy.

- The end-tidal CO_2 will rise during the course of a prolonged procedure and minute volume should be adjusted to compensate.
- Pneumothorax and surgical emphysema have been described, again associated with prolonged surgery.
- Caval compression and reduced venous return, with lowered cardiac output, may be a consequence of intra-abdominal pressure exceeding 4 kPa. The pressure effect of the insufflating gas will also splint the diaphragm and impede the mechanism of breathing.
- Shoulder-tip pain, from diaphragmatic irritation, is a common postoperative problem.

The laryngeal mask is widely used in gynaecological laparoscopy. Its use in laparoscopic cholecystectomy is contentious but some reports of this usage have been published. It is not recommended.

―――――――――――

EXAMPLE 9

Scenario
You are called to see an 18-year-old motorcyclist in A & E. He has been involved in an RTA and has obvious deformity of his right thigh and a scalp wound. How do you proceed?

⊃ **ABC first – as always. A quick estimation of the GCS and action as appropriate. You are told that he is alert, in pain and can move all four limbs. The immediate course of action is therefore:**

- Oxygen by face mask
- Assess cervical spine
- Caridovascular monitoring
- Fluid resuscitation (assume fractured femur)
- Assess blood loss from scalp
- Pain relief – consider femoral nerve block
- Bloods and X-rays appropriate to the results of primary survey

It is most likely that you will directed to choosing an appropriate technique for taking the patient to theatre for nailing of his femur. Rapid sequence induction followed by IPPV with volatile and opioid (maybe femoral block) is appropriate. Beware pneumothorax and hidden abdominal bleeding in any trauma scenario. Discuss the blood loss element with respect to adequate resuscitation pre-induction. Discuss the head-injury aspect, although this is not significant in the facts as given above.

Often this scenario leads onto a related critical incident. Occasionally, it is complicated by the fact that the victim has had breakfast and long acting insulin one hour prior to the accident.

CRITICAL INCIDENT – FAT EMBOLISM

The above patient is on table and his femur is being reamed. You are told that there is a sudden drop in end-tidal CO_2 concentration accompanied by desaturation and hypotension with an increase in airway pressure.

⊃ **You should say that embolism is most likely and it is probable that this will be a fat embolism, given the circumstances.**

Immediate management involves:
- 100% oxygen (bear in mind need for maintaining anaesthesia)
- Cardiovascular support
- Consider drugs – steroids, aprotinin, prostacyclin
- Prolonge IPPV may be necessary
- ITU care post-operatively
- May get ARDS and mortality approaches 10%

Other causes may be brought into discussion and should be approached systematically. Remember also that embolism of air, blood clot and cement can occur during orthopaedic procedures.

FURTHER CLINICAL TOPIC

How is blood cross-matched?

> ⊃ **Antigens present on red cell membranes. Mendelian inheritance applies to these antigens. There are two main groups for matching: the ABO system and Rhesus factor system.**

ABO system

Blood grouped for transfusion by the presence of antigens A, B, AB or absence (Group O) on the red cell surface.

If A or B antigen is absent then the opposite antibody (agglutinin) is present in the circulation

BLOOD TYPE	INCIDENCE IN THE UK	GENOTYPE	ANTIGEN (AGGLUTINOGENS)	ANTIBODIES (AGGLUTININS)
O	47%	OO	none	Anti- A, Anti- B
A	41%	OA, AA	A	Anti-B
B	9%	OB, BB	B	Anti-A
AB	3%	AB	A, B	none

Blood typing is a process of mixing the patient's blood sample with plasma that contains Anti-A or Anti-B agglutinins. Agglutination occurs if the samples are not compatible.

Cross-matching is the procedure that determines a patient's blood compatibility with the donor's red blood cells and plasma.

- Rhesus factor comprises C, D and E antigens
- Rh positive means that the D antigen is present (83% of population)
- The function of the D antigen is unknown
- Rh negative means that there is no D antigen. If an Rh-negative patient is injected with D positives, anti-D antibodies develop. Unlike the ABO system, the patient only develops agglutinins to D with exposure.

There are many other types of antigens (e.g. MN, Lutheran, Kell)

Chances of compatibility

No cross match   64%
ABO matched   99.4% (group specific)
ABO and Rhesus done   99.8%

A likely further question is: Are ABO antigens only found on red cells?

White cells and platelets carry some antigens which are also found on red cells, ABO, and MN for example but not the rhesus system.

These ABO antigens are also found as glycolipid, which is an alcohol soluble component of all body tissues (except the brain and spinal cord).

78% of individuals are "secretors" that is, they have the same antigens that correspond to the ABO system in a water-soluble form in saliva, urine and sweat.

EXAMPLE 10

Scenario

A 16-year-old boy is brought in to A & E from a nightclub by his friends. He is unrousable and the story appears to be that of a sudden collapse on leaving the club at 2 AM. You are crash bleeped to attend the admission. How will you proceed?

⊃ **ABC straight away – You are told he is breathing by the examiner and also cardiovascularly stable. The priority then is to assess the conscious level.**

■ **AVPU**

■ **GCS**

are both appropriate. Are there any pupillary signs? You may be asked for details of AVPU and GCS.

A brief outline follows:
The AVPU scale for rapid neurological assessment

A   Alert

V   Responds to vocal stimuli

P   Responds to painful stimuli

U   Unresponsive

Glasgow Coma Scale

BEST PERFORMANCE	SCORE
Eye opening	
Spontaneous	4
To speech	3
To pain	2
Nil	1
Verbal response	
Oriented	5
Confused	4
Inappropriate	3
Incomprehensible	2
Nil	1
Motor response	
Obeying commands	5
Localising	4
Flexing	3
Extending	2
Nil	1

If GCS is less than 5, consider intubation. Discuss the benefits and risks of this in the context of the uncertain diagnosis. If airway reflexes are absent the airway **must** be secured. Likely diagnoses:

- Drugs – alcohol and psychotropics (any clues?)
- Intracranial event
- Metabolic causes
- Head trauma

Uncertainty over the cause will be elucidated by clinical examination, blood tests and CAT scan. Discuss the problems of transport and monitoring in scanners.

CRITICAL INCIDENT – HYPOTENSION

You are called by the ward nurses to see a post operative hip replacement patient whose blood pressure is 80/40 on an automatic machine. They are concerned. What is your approach?

> ⊃ **The commonest cause is hypovolaemia and this should be considered before other factors, though they may co-exist. You should therefore immediately assess blood loss (anaesthetic record, drains, pallor, tachycardia) and organise colloid resuscitation and oxygen by face mask if this is the likely cause.**

After the initial stabilisation of the patient you will probably be asked about the various causes of hypotension. Structure your answer according to the physiological and pharmacological factors that affect blood pressure:

Venous return
A. Hypovolaemia
- inadequate intra-operative fluid replacement
- bleeding either overt or concealed

B. Postural changes

C. Tension pneumothorax

D. Cardiac tamponade

E. Aorto-caval compression
- Pregnancy
- Large intra-abdominal mass

Systemic vascular resistance
A. Warming leading to vasodilation and relative hypovolaemia

B. Anaesthetic agents
- Inhalational and intravenous agents
- Spinal or epidural anaesthesia
- Opioids

C. Hypotensive agents given pre- and intra-operatively

D. Spinal cord trauma

Myocardial function

A. Arrhythmias

B. Myocardial ischaemia or infarction

C. Left ventricular failure

Others

A. Cushing's syndrome

B. Myxoedema

C. Intracranial pathology

FURTHER CLINICAL TOPIC

Under what circumstances might additional corticosteroids be necessary?

> ⊃ **To answer this question, break your response into what steroids do, what happens during surgery and why they need to be administered during surgery.**

Normal actions of steroids include an increase in plasma glucose by promoting substrate breakdown and gluconeogenesis, immune modulation and anti-inflammatory action, fluid retention, and inhibition of the actions of interleukins.

When confronted by the stress of major surgery, plasma cortisol concentrations increase within 4 hours and remain elevated for up to 3 days after surgery. The daily production may increase from the base line of 25 mg of cortisol per day up to 500 mg per day. Where adrenal function is suppressed by the administration of exogenous steroids, this response to the stress of surgery may not occur and the features of an Addisonian crisis may become apparent. This will include:

- Hypoglycaemia
- Hypotension
- Hypovolaemia
- Hyperkalaemia
- Hyponatraemia

Patients at risk of this are those patients who are taking long-term glucocorticoid medication. This may be by the oral, parenteral and possibly inhaled routes. Fluticazone has been implicated in adrenal suppression at a dose of less than 1 mg a day. However, patients taking less than 10 mg of prednisolone a day are regarded as having a normal adrenal response. Where patients have stopped taking glucocorticoids more than 3 months previously it is assumed that their stress response is back to normal; however those patients who have been taking steroids within the previous 3 months should be considered to be at risk. Current recommendations include the administration of 25 mg of hydrocortisone at induction of anaesthesia in addition to the patient's usual glucocorticoid intake. For moderate and major surgery a 100 mg of hydrocortisone should be administered daily for 3 to 4 days. It is no longer regarded as necessary to reduce the supplementation incrementally.

———————————————

EXAMPLE 11

Scenario

The first patient on your gynaecology list, scheduled for a total abdominal hysterectomy, tells you that when she had her gall bladder out she was told 'They had trouble getting the tube in'. How would you assess her airway?

> ⊃ **Although many practitioners would use an LMA, assume you are being directed towards an assessment of intubating conditions – unless told otherwise by the examiner.**

Clinical assessment of the airway is essential. Start with gross observations (Fat neck? No chin?). In the Mallampati scoring system the patient sits opposite the anaesthetist with mouth open and tongue protruded. The structures visible at the back of the mouth are noted (Mallampati 1985) as described below.

- **Class 1** – Faucial pillars, soft palate and uvula visible
- **Class 2** – Faucial pillars and soft palate visible, uvula masked by base of tongue
- **Class 3** – Only soft palate visible
- **Class 4** – Soft palate not visible

The modified Mallampati classification produces a high incidence of false positives. If the thyromental distance with the neck extended is less than 6.5 cm or the width of three fingers, difficult intubation is predicted. A thyromental distance of less than 6.5 cm and Mallampati class 3 or 4 predicts 80% of difficult intubations.

The Wilson risk factors may provide additional predictive information on the airway. The Wilson risk factors each score 0–2 points, to give a maximum of 10 points. A score > 2 predicts 75% of difficult intubations, also with a high incidence of false positives. The Wilson risk factors are:

- Obesity
- Restricted head and neck movements
- Restricted jaw movement
- Receding mandible
- Buck teeth

Inability to flex the chin onto the chest indicates poor neck movement. Once the neck is fully flexed, a patient should be able to move their head more than 15° to demonstrate normal occipito-axial movement. Reduced jaw movements are demonstrated by poor mouth opening (particularly if of less than two fingers' width) and by inability to protrude the lower teeth beyond the upper.

Radiological features may aid prediction of a difficult intubation but are not routinely performed. They include:

- Reduced distance between occiput and spine of C1 and between spines of C1 and C2

- Ratio of mandibular length to posterior mandibular depth > 3.6
- Increased depth of mandible

This line of questioning may lead to a discussion of difficult intubation. Ease of intubation has been graded according to the best possible view obtained on laryngoscopy (Cormack 1984). Grades 3 and 4 are difficult intubations.

- **Grade 1** – Whole of glottis visible
- **Grade 2** – Glottis incompletely visible
- **Grade 3** – Epiglottis but not glottis visible
- **Grade 4** – Epiglottis not visible

The reported incidence of difficult intubation varies, but is around 1 in 65 intubations. Despite careful history and examination, 20% of difficult intubations are not predicted. The consequences may be disastrous. A history of previous difficult intubation is important but a history of straightforward intubation several years earlier may be falsely reassuring. As the patient's weight, cervical spine movement and disease process may all have changed. Some congenital conditions may predict a difficult intubation e.g. Pierre Robin syndrome, Marfan's syndrome or cystic hygroma. Pathological conditions can make intubation difficult e.g. tumour, infection or scarring of the upper airway tissues. There is no one test that is able to predict all difficult intubations.

CRITICAL INCIDENT – MALIGNANT HYPERTHERMIA

A patient on table is demonstrating a fast rise in temperature and you suspect the devlopment of malignant hyperthermia. How will you proceed?

> ⟳ **Keep this practical. The discussion of the pathophysiology of MH is usually covered in the further clinical topic – see below. This is about the management of a suspected case.**

FIRST – CALL FOR HELP

Primary management
Stop the use of all MH trigger agents. Change the anaesthesia machine; and change from the circle system, if it is being used, to a non-rebreathing system. Terminate surgery if possible. Monitor the ECG and capnograph. Alert the intensive care unit. Commence invasive monitoring. Delegate one person to prepare dantrolene sodium 1 mg/kg. Record core temperature, pulse rate and blood pressure every 5 min. Measure arterial pH and blood gases. Treat hypercarbia with vigorous hyperventilation, acidosis with sodium bicarbonate 2–4 mmol/kg. Maintain oxygenation. Save one venous sample for serum CK and send one for electrolytes and serum calcium estimations. Give IV dantrolene sodium 1 mg/kg. Repeat at 10 minute intervals if necessary, up to a maximum of 10 mg/kg.

Secondary management
Cool the patient and keep the first urine sample for myoglobin estimation. Measure urine output. If obvious myoglobinuria occurs, give intravenous fluids, and mannitol or frusemide to promote urine flow. The use of steroids is controversial, but may be indicated for cerebral oedema in the severe case. Repeat the serum CK

estimation at 24 hours. Treat DIC if necessary. Dantrolene may need to be repeated for up to 24 hours as retriggering may occur.

FURTHER CLINICAL TOPIC

What do you understand by the term 'Malignant Hyperthermia'?

> ⊃ **You will only have time for a limited discussion on this huge topic, so try and be succinct. *Treatment* is usually confined to the critical incident, so use a more structured general answer in this section.**

MH is exceedingly rare but of great importance to the anaesthetist. The mortality in the 1970s was 70% or more and although today it is closer to 25%. The reduction in mortality probably reflects an increased awareness of the condition, more intensive patient monitoring for sensitive indicators, such as end tidal carbon dioxide tension, which assist early diagnosis; and the availability of an intravenous form of dantrolene sodium, a drug which has played an important role in the treatment of MH.

Pathophysiology

MH may represent a spectrum of conditions rather than a specific pharmacogenetic entity as the inheritance is complex. Presentation under anaesthesia is usually that of a marked increase in metabolic rate arising from accelerated muscle metabolism. At cellular level the exact defect remains unclear but dysfunction of the sarcoplasmic reticulum and abnormalities of intracellular ionic calcium transport occur, with a secondary effect of increased sympathetic nervous system activity. Agents known to induce MH cause an enhanced release of calcium from the sarcoplasmic reticulum and a generalised membrane permeability defect develops. Genetic studies indicate that the MH gene is on chromosome 19, in a position close to the ryanodine receptor gene. Features of MH are given below.

Features of MH

Cardinal physical signs
- Hyperthermia (core temperature rising by a minimum of 1–2 °C/H)
- Respiratory acidosis (hypercarbia)
- Metabolic acidosis (with or without muscle rigidity)
- Cardiac arrhythmias
- Hypoxaemia
- Cyanosis (from a large rise in oxygen consumption plus ventilation perfusion defects)

Signs of abnormal muscle activity
- Failure of the jaw to relax after suxamethonium
- Rigidity of certain, but not necessarily of all, groups of muscles.
- Hyperkalaemia
- Myoglobinuria and renal failure
- Rise in creatinine kinase

Other signs
- Disseminated intravascular coagulation (DIC)
- Cerebral and pulmonary oedema

Triggering agents
ALL the inhalational agents including desflurane and sevoflurane suxamethonium (avoid if possible-phenothiazines, atropine)

Agents thought to be safe
- Thiopentone
- Propofol
- Nitrous oxide
- Opioids
- Pancuronium
- Vecuronium
- Benzodiazepines
- Amide local anaesthetics

EXAMPLE 12

Scenario
A 77-year-old previously fit lady is admitted following a fall at home. She has sustained a fractured neck of femur and you are asked to anaesthetise her for hip screws. What information is important?

⊃ **Consider head injury, reason for the fall – cardiac event? neurological event? Consider urgency of operation – probably able to wait for investigations and optimaisation. Past medical history? Usual pre anaesthetic checks –medication, allergies, previous surgery.**

Request Hb, U and E, Glucose, CXR, ECG. Assuming these are normal the questioning will often turn to a choice of GA vs RA. There is little difference in long term mortality between them (over 3 months).

Contraindications to RA: Infection, neurological disease, anticoagulation, deformity of spine, patient refusal.

The examiner may lead you into choosing a spinal as the technique for this lady. You may be asked about spinal needle design and headache incidence and the anatomy of the layers through which you pass as you perform a spinal. Management of this case should include the avoidance of hypotension and consideration of sedation.

Make sure you can deal safely with a 'total spinal'. This clinical scenario is often blended with a total spinal as the critical incident component of the viva in a seamless manner!

CRITICAL INCIDENT – ANAPHYLAXIS

You are giving a test dose of cefuroxime to an elderly man prior to inducing anaesthesia for his hip replacement. He says he is having trouble breathing, starts to wheeze and you think his eyes are closing up due to swelling. What do you do?

⊃ **Suggest a diagnosis of anaphylaxis and stop the injection first of all.**

The prompt and aggressive treatment of a patient with a severe anaphylactic reaction is life saving. Administer 100% oxygen and consider early intubation before the onset of angio-oedema. The administration of adrenaline is a priority, and if there is circulatory collapse 1ml of 1 in 10 000 adrenaline should be administered IV at 1 minute intervals. Intravenous colloids are the most effective treatment to restore intravascular volume, up to two litres may be infused rapidly (note that allergic reaction to colloids administered at this time is virtually unknown). Arrhythmias should be treated symptomatically. Bronchospasm can be difficult to overcome and although adrenaline is often effective aminophylline and nebulised salbutamol may be useful for persistent bronchospasm. Intratracheal injections of local anaesthetic agents (such as lidocaine 100 mg) have also been advocated. Although such reactions are rare all anaesthetists should rehearse a simulated 'anaphylaxis drill' at regular intervals. See below.

Management of a patient with suspected anaphylaxis

(Association of Anaesthetists – Suspected anaphylactic reactions associated with anaesthesia, 1995).

Initial therapy

1. Stop administration of drug(s) likely to be responsible
2. Maintain airway-give 100% oxygen
3. Lay patient flat with feet elevated
4. Give adrenaline
   IM   0.5 mg to 1.0 mg and repeated every 10 minutes as required
   IV   50 to 100 mcg over 1 minute and repeated as required
   For cardiovascular collapse 0.5 to 1.0 mg (5 to 10 ml of 1 in 10 000) may be required intravenously in divided doses by titration. This should be given at a rate of 0.1 mg (1 ml of 1 in 10 000) per minute until a response is obtained.
5. Start intravascular volume expansion with crystalloid or colloid

Secondary therapy

1. Antihistamines (chlorpheniramine 10–20 mg by slow intravenous infusion)
2. Corticosteriods (100–300 mg hydrocortisone iv)
3. Catecholamine infusions consider: adrenaline   4–8 mcg / min
                                         noradrenaline   4–8 mcg / min
4. Consider bicarbonate 0.5–1.0 mg/kg IV for acidosis
5. Airway evaluation (before extubation)
6. Bronchodilators may be required for persistent bronchospasm.

Follow up

After a suspected drug reaction associated with anaesthesia the patient should be counselled and investigated. This is the responsibility of the anaesthetist who administered the drug and should be conducted in consultation with a clinical immunologist. No tests or investigations of any kind should be performed until the resuscitation period is completed. Approximately one hour after the reaction occurred 10 ml of venous blood should be taken into a plain glass tube, the serum separated and stored at –20°C for estimation of serum tryptase concentration. Elevation of this enzyme indicates that the reaction was associated with mast cell degranulation. Blood samples in EDTA containing tubes are useful for complement assays and haematology; the disappearance of basophils being indicative of a Type 1 anaphylactic reaction. When more than one drug has been administered skin prick tests are useful to establish the agent involved. These should be carried out by specialised departments with full resuscitation facilities.

FURTHER CLINICAL TOPIC

What are the indications for tracheal intubation?

> ⊃ **These may be divided into protection of the upper airway, protection of the lower airway, and where paralysis is required for other reasons.**

1. Protection of the upper airway, when ENT surgeons or facial surgeons are at work in the nose and mouth. This is also known as "the shared airway".
2. Protection of the lower airway, in other words, prevention of aspiration of gastric contents where there is a full stomach, an acute abdomen, and in obstetrics. Where there is cardiovascular collapse, intubation and ventilation is usual.
3. Where muscle relaxation is required, for surgery (and ventilation also, therefore) or it is a prolonged procedure, when atelectasis might occur with prolonged spontaneous respiration.

The discussion may lead on from this to the types of equipment needed and the variety of ET tubes that are available and their various indications.

EXAMPLE 13

Scenario
The first patient on your gynaecology list (for hysteroscopy) tells you she is allergic to latex. What do you know about latex allergy?

⊃ **This is a general question that can be answered with a general overview. It is likely, however that the questioning will proceed on to the precautions necessary when anaesthetising latex sensitive patients.**

You should begin by saying that allergy to natural rubber latex is an increasing problem for health care workers who may have to carry out procedures on patients who react to latex or who may themselves develop reactions to latex. The reactions tend to fall into two groups, either skin contact or anaphylactic in type. Both are serious problems and no distinction should be made between them.

Natural latex contains a variety of highly allergenic proteins, which cause reaction by repeated exposure and hypersensitivity. Continued exposure increases the severity of the reaction. It is interesting that there are reports of cross-reactions to similar proteins in fruits such as banana, avocado and kiwi fruit as well as nuts.

If a patient reports possible latex allergy then, while skin testing by dermatologists is possible, it is time consuming and potentially dangerous so it may be wise to accept the patient at face value and treat them as if they are positive. Many latex sensitive patients will have a history of skin reactions to rubber gloves, condoms or balloons.

What special precautions would you take?
- For planned surgery the patient should be first on a morning operating list to avoid the possibility of latex particles being in the operating theatre atmosphere.
- All staff should be familiar with the local latex allergy policy and aware of their responsibilities. Traffic in the room should be kept to a minimum.
- All staff should wear non-latex gloves.
- If possible all anaesthetic breathing system tubing should be made of plastics or man-made rubbers such as neoprene. If it is not possible to replace this tubing then it should be covered with stockinet gauze to prevent transfer of particles from the rubber to the patient by staff handling the exposed rubber.
- Blood pressure cuff bladders and tubing should be covered so that there is no contact with the patient.
- All breathing systems should have a bacterial filter at the patient end to prevent latex particles entering the patient's airway.
- For airway maintenance PVC tracheal tubes and laryngeal mask airways are acceptable, as they do not contain latex. Facemasks should be made of plastic.

IV-V cannulae are usually latex-free though it is always wise to check beforehand. Syringes should be checked for latex, though most modern syringes are latex-free and labelled as such.

Standard blood giving sets contain latex in the injection port at the cannula connection. These should be avoided. Even supposedly latex-free fluid giving sets may contain latex in injection ports. These should be removed but if this is not possible, should not be used as injection ports because of the possibility of coring and embolising particles of latex. A three-way tap is preferable. The rubber seals on drug ampoules do not contain latex. Equipment for local and regional anaesthesia does not usually contain latex but each anaesthetic department should identify which products are latex-free and keep a stock of these products. There are lists of latex-free and latex-containing products on the internet at ***www.immune. com/rubber/ukdatabase***.

An anaphylaxis pack should be available in the operating theatre while a latex-allergic patient is present. The patient should be anaesthetised in the operating theatre and recover in the same room rather than being transferred to a recovery room where the atmosphere is less well controlled. Each anaesthetic and operating theatre department should develop a policy on the management of latex allergy and a box containing latex-free equipment. All staff should familiarise themselves with both of these.

CRITICAL INCIDENT – BRADYCARDIA

You proceed with anaesthesia on this patient and while the cervix is being dilated you notice an extreme drop in heart rate, down to 30 bpm. How do you react?

⊃ **Put yourself in the real situation. This requires action, not theory.**

Firstly stop the surgeon. Instruments out and leave the patient entirely alone. Then:

- Remove volatile and nitrous oxide
- Hand ventilate with 100% oxygen
- Prepare and administer a vagolytic drug if heart rate remains low (glycopyrrollate is preferable as atropine has a biphasic effect and thus may initially make things worse due to a central nervous system effect)
- Consider CPM if the situation does not improve
- If asystole develops a suitable algorithm should be instituted

This critical incident appears frequently in the examination and is not always answered well.

What are the causes of bradycardia under anaesthesia?

The most important cause of bradycardia under anaesthesia is hypoxia. It may also be due to surgical, drug-related, metabolic or disease-related causes.

Surgical
1. Manual dilatation of the anus
2. Eye and orbit procedures
3. Laparoscopy
4. Laparotomy with mesenteric traction
5. Dilation of the cervix

Drugs
1. Halothane.
2. Neostigmine.
3. Suxamethonium, with special reference to the second dose.
4. Spinal blockade at T1-T4, which is seen in Spinal anaesthesia and spinal injuries.

Metabolic
1. Hypothyroidism.
2. Hyperkalaemia.

Disease
1. Ischaemic heart disease.
2. Raised intracranial pressure.

FURTHER CLINICAL TOPIC

How is blood stored?

All donated blood starts as 450 ml from the donor, with 60 ml additive, cooled to 4°C.

There are two main types of blood admixture, CAPD and SAGM.

CAPD = citrate, adenine, phosphate, dextrose
SAGM = sodium chloride, adenine, glucose, mannitol
  ▪ Random blood has a chance of 64.0%   compatibility
  ▪ An ABO cross match   99.4%   compatibility
  ▪ ABO and rhesus cross match   99.8%   compatibility
  ▪ Full cross match   99.95% compatibility

UK plasma is burnt due to the risk of transmitting spongiform encephalopathy due to prions (ridiculously low) and plasma is imported, mostly from the USA.

Stored blood has pH 6.9, K^+ 20 mmol/l, HCO_3^- 10 mmol/l.

Mention if time allows that the filters in giving sets are 180 µm whereas depth or screen types are ususlly 20 or 40 µm pore size.

EXAMPLE 14

Scenario

You are presented with a 62-year-old man for elective repair of an inguinal hernia. He has always smoked 20+ a day since the age of 14 and has a persistent cough. He denies any other medical problems. The patient asks you if a spinal anaesthetic would be suitable as his friend recently had one. Do you think this is a suitable technique for this patient?

⊃ **This requires a clinical approach. Take the history, examine, consider.**

Begin by getting more detail about the bronchitis, which will surely be present. Sputum, antibiotic use, visits to GP, wheezing and any history of haemoptysis.

Ask for examination findings – likely to have widespread ronchi and perhaps wheeze throughout. Are there any vitalograph results? You may be shown one.

Assuming no acute infection or other complications check next for any contraindications to spinal anaesthesia. Consider:

- Anticoagulation
- Hypotensive medication
- Spinal deformity
- Previous laminectomy
- Difficult airway
- Inability to lie flat

In the absence of contraindications a spinal technique is entirely suitable for a hernia repair if an in patient bed is available. Expect to be asked about the practical technique, needle choice, block height, drugs. Do not forget to administer oxygen on the table and be cautious in patients with respiratory compromise when choosing to sedate or not. Benzodiazepines are particularly unpredictable in their respiratory depressant effects.

CRITICAL INCIDENT – NEEDLE STICK

You inadvertently pierce you hand with a used cannula when inducing a fit 20-year-old for extraction of wisdom teeth. What are the procedures required?

Following injury, the puncture site should be encouraged to bleed vigorously and thoroughly washed with soap and water. Eye splashes should be rinsed with sterile eye-wash or water.

Occupational exposure must be reported and recorded in an accident book. Each unit may have a different protocol for this, but most require attendance at A and E. Blood should be taken from the victim, and in high risk scenarios from the patient (after appropriate consent). If after consideration of the relative risk (taking into account HIV and hepatitis status) prophylaxis is considered desirable this should be instituted. Triple therapy is usual and this comprises three antiviral drugs, a combination of protease inhibitors and nucleoside analogue reverse transcriptase inhibitors. Counselling should be made available through the occupational health department.

Note: Infection with the human immunodeficiency virus was only recognised in 1983 but there must have been numerous unrecognised cases before that. The virus is delicate, easily destroyed and has low infectivity. The main routes of transmission are by promiscuous sexual activity (both heterosexual and homosexual) and by the sharing of injection equipment. Many haemophiliacs have been infected by pooled blood transfusion products which were drawn from an infected community before the problem was recognised. Needle stick injury is not a major route of infection except in the case of a large innoculate or frequent small innoculation from an infected population, such as when performing surgery in sub-Saharan Africa. HIV and Hepatitis B frequently occur together, particularly in prostitutes and in the homosexual and drug abusing communities.

FURTHER CLINICAL TOPIC

What precautions should you take to prevent a patient under anaesthesia from coming to harm through non-surgical causes?

- Care when positioning on the table
- Protection of the eyes especially prone position
- Lips, teeth, crowns – avoidance of trauma
- If tying in ETT not too tight
- Skin care, padding where pressure points exist
- Nerve injuries (*see diagram*)
- Cervical spine, hips, jaw – avoid unnecessary force
- Warm fluids and patient
- Appropriate diathermy plate siting

The more common nerves to consider and the positions that make them vulnerable are shown in the diagram (overleaf).

Position	Nerve injury	Cause
	supra-orbital	pressure from an endotracheal tube connector
	nerves innervating the eyeball	pressure by a face mask
SUPINE	cranial nerve VII	pressure by a tight face mask harness
	brachial plexus	traction injury due to incorrect positioning or from shoulder retainers in the Trendelenberg position
	radial nerve	pressure by screen supports
	ulnar nerve	pressure by the edge of the operating table mattress

Position	Nerve injury	Cause
	cervical spine	movement up or down the operating table
	sciatic nerve	stretching of nerve between sciatic notch and neck of fibula
LITHOTOMY as above plus	femoral nerve	flexion of thigh may stretch nerve against ingunal ligament
	posterior tibial nerve	pressure from stirrups
	common peroneal nerve	compression against head of fibula
	saphenous nerve	compression against the medial tibial condyle
	obturator nerve	flexion at the obturator foramen

Position	Nerve injury	Cause
	cervical spinal cord	over extension of the cervical spine
	brachial plexus	overdistension
PRONE	radial nerve	direct compression
	ulnar nerve	compression at the elbow against a mattress
	LCNT	pressure on the anterior superior iliac spine

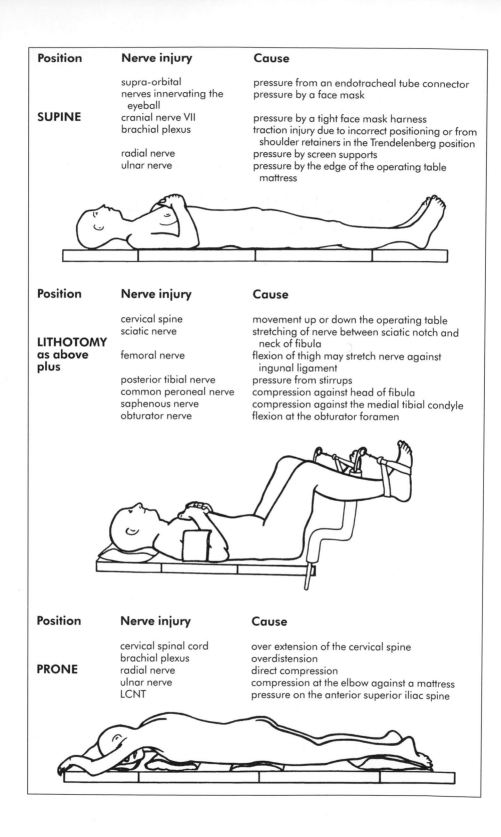

APPENDIX 1

USEFUL DEFINITIONS AND FORMULAE IN PHYSICS

Mathematics and Units

A general quadratic function **is expressed as:**

$$y = Ax^2 + Bx + C$$

An **exponential function** can be written in two ways:

$$y = A \exp(-kt) \text{ or } y = A e^{-kt}$$

The Time constant is expressed as: $\dfrac{1}{K}$

and this is related to the half life by:

$$\text{Half life} = 0.693 \times \text{time constant}$$

Common Integrals

Function f(t)	Integral
1	t
t	$\dfrac{t^2}{2}$
t^2	$\dfrac{t^3}{3}$
exp (at)	$\dfrac{1}{a}$ exp (at)
sin (at)	$\dfrac{-1}{a}$ cos (at)
cos (at)	$\dfrac{1}{a}$ sin (at)

Common Derivatives

Function $f(t)$	Derivative
t	1
t^2	2t
t^3	$3t^2$
exp (at)	a. exp (at)
sin (at)	a. cos (at)
cos (at)	$-$ a. sin (at)

Fundamental units and supplementary units in the SI system

Quantity	Unit	Symbol
Length	metre	m
Mass	kilogram	kg
Time	second	s
Electric current	ampere	A
Temperature	kelvin	K
Amount of substance (specify particles e.g. atoms, molecules, ions)	mole	mol
Light intensity	candela	cd

Supplementary Units

Angle	radian	rad
Solid angle	steradian	sr

Derived SI units

Phenomenon	Derived Unit	Symbol
Area	square metre	m^2
Volume	cubic metre	m^3
Density	kilogram per cubic metre	kg/m^3
Velocity	metre per second	m/s
Acceleration	metre per second per second	m/s^2

Named derived units

Phenomenon	Derived Unit	Name (Symbol)	Unit Description
Force	$kg.m/s^2$	newton (N)	Force required to accelerate a mass of one kg at 1 m/s^2
Pressure	$kg/m.s^2$	pascal (Pa)	Pressure which exerts a force of 1 newton per square metre of surface area
Frequency	$1/s$	hertz (Hz)	Number of cycles of a periodic activity per second
Energy	$kg.m^2/s^2$	joule (J)	Energy expended in moving a resistive force of 1 newton a distance of 1 metre
Power	$kg.m^2/s^3$	watt (W)	Rate of energy expenditure of 1 joule per second

Prefixes used to denote unit multiplication factors

Prefix	Letter	Multiplying factor
exa	E	10^{18}
peta	P	10^{15}
tera	T	10^{12}
giga	G	10^{9}
mega	M	10^{6}
kilo	k	10^{3}
hecto	h	$10^{?}$
decca	da	10
deci	d	10^{-1}
centi	h	10^{-2}
milli	m	10^{-3}
micro	μ	10^{-6}
nano	n	10^{-9}
pico	p	10^{-12}
femto	f	10^{-15}
atto	a	10^{-18}

Conversion between atmospheric pressure units

Basic unit	Converted equivalent	
1.0 kPa	1000	N/m^2
	0.01	bar
	0.01013	atmospheres
	10^4	$dyne/cm^2$
	7.5	mmHg
	10.2	cmH_2O
	0.145	pounds force per square inch
	20.9	pounds force per square foot

FUNDAMENTAL CONSTANTS

These are basic constants, which have internationally agreed values. An example is the speed of light in a vacuum, which is now given the value of 299792458 m/s. This enables the unit of length to be defined. The metre is now defined as the length of the path travelled by light in a vacuum during a time interval of 1/299792458 of a second.

Other fundamental constants include the elementary charge of an electron (1.602×10^{-19} C), the Faraday constant (9.648×10^4 C/mol), Avogadro's number (6.022×10^{23}) and the Gas Constant (R).

Humidity

Commonly used temperature scales showing freezing and boiling points of water

Scale	Freezing Point H_2O	Boiling Point H_2O
Kelvin	273.15	373.15
Celsius	0	100
Fahrenheit	32	212

Absolute humidity: Mass of water vapour present in a given volume of air. The units of measurement are grams per cubic metre (g/m^3) or kilograms per cubic metre (kg/m^3). Absolute humidity value will not vary with the temperature of the air.

Relative humidity: Ratio of the mass of water present in a given volume of air at a given temperature, to the mass of water required to saturate that given volume at the same temperature. Relative humidity is usually expressed as a percentage, and it varies with temperature.

GASES

The Three Gas Laws

1. The relationship between volume and pressure at constant temperature is described by Boyle's law:

Pressure is inversely proportional to volume

$$P \quad \propto \quad \frac{1}{V}$$

or $\quad$ PV $\quad = \quad$ constant

2. The relationship between volume and temperature at constant pressure is described by Charles' law:

Volume is proportional to temperature (degrees Kelvin)

$$V \quad \propto \quad T$$

or $\quad$ VT $\quad = \quad$ constant

3. The relationship between pressure and temperature at constant volume is described by Gay-Lussac's law:

Pressure is proportional to temperature (degrees Kelvin)

$$P \quad \propto \quad T$$

or $\quad$ PT $\quad = \quad$ constant

The above three laws can be summarised into a single equation, the Ideal Gas Equation:

$$\frac{PV}{T} \quad = \quad constant$$

This equation enables conversion from one set of conditions to another when a fixed mass of gas undergoes changes in pressure, volume or temperature, since:

$$\frac{P_1V_1}{T_1} \quad = \quad \frac{P_2V_2}{T_1}$$

The gas constant (R)

The ideal gas equation may be written as:

$$PV \quad = \quad kT$$

where k is a constant dependent on the mass of gas present, if n = number of moles of gas present, the Ideal Gas Equation becomes:

$$PV \quad = \quad nRT$$

where **R** is known as the Universal Gas Constant, and can be evaluated by considering 1 mole of gas at 273K (0°C) at a pressure of 1 atmosphere. This gives a value of **R** = 8.32 joules per °C

Dalton's law of partial pressures

This states that if a mixture of gases is placed in a container then the pressure exerted by each gas (partial pressure) is equal to that which it would exert if it alone occupied the container

Hagen-Poiseuille law

Hagen (in 1839) and Poiseuille (in 1840) discovered the laws governing laminar flow through a tube. If a pressure P is applied across the ends of a tube of length, l, and radius, r. Then the flow rate, Q, produced is proportional to:

- The pressure gradient (P/l)
- The fourth power of the tube radius (r^4)
- The reciprocal of fluid viscosity ($1/\eta$)

This is often combined as:

$$Q = \frac{\pi\, P\, r^4}{8\,\eta\, l}$$

and attributed to Poiseuille, a surgeon, who verified this relationship experimentally.

Reynold's number

The Reynolds number (Re) is used to determine whether the flow will be laminar or turbulent in any given situation. It includes the kinematic viscosity, μ and the ratio of the inertial forces to the viscous damping forces in the fluid and is given by:

$$Re = \frac{v\, l}{\mu}$$

Where v = the mean flow velocity for flow through a tube, or the velocity a long way from an object. l = a characteristic length of the system, such as the diameter of a tube.

At low Reynolds numbers, the viscous forces dampen minor irregularities in the flow, resulting in a laminar pattern. A high Reynolds number means that the inertial forces dominate, and any eddies in the flow will be easily created and persist for a long time, creating turbulence. For flow though a tube, a Reynolds number of less than 2000 tends to give laminar flow, while between 2000 and 4000, the flow may be a mixture of laminar and turbulent depending on the smoothness of the fluid entering the tube. Above 4000, the flow will certainly be turbulent.

ELECTRICITY

Ohm's law

Ohm's law states that the current flowing through a resistance is proportional to the potential difference across it. Potential difference across the resistance = V volts, current = I amps and the resistance has a value of R Ω.

So:

$$V = I\,R \quad \text{volts}$$

The flow of current through the resistance requires the expenditure of energy, which appears as heat. The power, P, dissipated as heat is given by:

$$P = VI \quad \text{watts}$$

Substituting for I or V, this may become:

$$P = I^2R \quad \text{watts}$$

$$= \frac{V^2}{R} \quad \text{watts}$$

Physiological effects at different current levels in AC mains shock

CURRENT (mA)	EFFECTS
0 – 5	Tingling sensation
5 – 10	Pain
10 – 50	Severe pain Muscle spasm
50 – 100	Respiratory muscle spasm Ventricular fibrillation Myocardial failure

LIGHT

Snell's law, states that for light travelling between two given media (where c is the speed of light in the medium):

$$\frac{\sin i}{\sin r} = \frac{c_1}{c_2}$$

The refractive properties of a medium are measured by its absolute refractive index (n), which is defined by:

$$\text{refractive index (n)} = \frac{\text{speed of light in a vacuum (c)}}{\text{speed of light in medium } (c_1)}$$

Lambert – Bouguer law: When a layer of solution of known thickness (d), is transilluminated by monochromatic light, the transmitted light (I) is related to the incident light (I_O), by:

$$I = I_O e^{-(ad)}$$

Where (ad) is the 'absorbance' or 'optical density' of the layer of solution. This in turn is the product of its thickness (d) and the quantity (a) known as the extinction coefficient of the solution.

Beer's law: This states that for a solution absorbance is a linear function of molar concentration

Combining the above laws gives the **Lambert-Beer law,** which relates the transmitted light to both molar concentration and thickness of the solution layer by expressing the absorbance as:

Absorbance = ϵ c d

Where ϵ = molar extinction coefficient, c = molar concentration, d = thickness.

APPENDIX 2

EXAMPLES OF CRITICAL INCIDENT TOPICS

Sudden pneumothorax – on table or in trauma victim

Rise in temperature under anaesthesia – MH

Failure to breathe after laparotomy

Sudden bradycardia during surgery

Needlestick injury to oneself

Embolism – fat,clot,air,amniotic fluid or methacrylate cement

Rise in airway pressure during IPPV

Massive haemorrhage

Wrong blood transfusion

Anaphylactic reaction

Failure to intubate

Aspiration of stomach contents – on intubation, extubation or in recovery

Convulsions in recovery – not known epileptic patient

Desaturation during anaesthesia

Failure to reverse after paralysis

Acute ST changes on the ECG monitor during operation

Arrhythmias under anaesthesia – VE, VT, and VF

Total spinal

Sudden cyanosis – recovery and on table

Hypotension in recovery or on table

Hypertension in recovery or on table

INDEX

INDEX

Note: Page references in **bold** refer to the appendices.

THE HANLEY LIBRARY
AND INFORMATION CENTRE